SCARED SKINNY NO MORE!

Exposing the Myths of Weight Bias and Weight Loss

Dr. Brad Johnson
Mary Dimino

Scared Skinny No More!

For information about special discounts for bulk purchases, please contact Sunbury Press, Inc. Wholesale Dept. at (717) 254-7274 or orders@sunburypress.com.

To request one of our authors for speaking engagements or book signings, please contact Sunbury Press, Inc. Publicity Dept. at publicity@sunburypress.com.

FIRST SUNBURY PRESS EDITION
Printed in the United States of America
March 2013

Trade paperback ISBN: 978-1-62006-185-5
Mobipocket format (Kindle) ISBN: 978-1-62006-186-2
ePub format (Nook) ISBN: 978-1-62006-187-9

Published by:
Sunbury Press
Mechanicsburg, PA
www.sunburypress.com

SUNBURY PRESS

Mechanicsburg, Pennsylvania USA

Mary:

For the wonderful gifts of life and love,
I dedicate this book to my beautiful mother and grandmother, whose battles with weight and health have molded me into the person I am today.
I thank you.
Also to my father, whose unconditional love was a beacon in my darkest times. Although you are not here, you are always with me.

Brad:

To my mother, thank you for your constant support and encouragement. You have always been a role model with your grace, strength, and perseverance. You have influenced more lives than you will ever know. Thank you for everything.

Somewhere out beyond the ideas of
skinny and fat there is a field.
I'll meet you there.

Contents

Acknowledgments

This book is a culmination of not only what seems like a lifetime of research, but of people and experiences that have touched our hearts and minds.

It takes a village to write a book.

The authors gratefully acknowledge Lawrence Knorr at Sunbury Press, our dedicated editor Allyson Gard, Jeffrey Lyle Johnson, our gifted resident artist and everyone who has made this book possible and seen it through to its birth.

And thank *you* dear reader. May we discover each other more in every page.

About the Authors

Dr. Brad Johnson is author of *The Edutainer: Connecting the Art and Science of Teaching* (2010). Dr. Johnson has over 20 years experience in the wellness and fitness field. His degrees include a bachelor's degree in wellness, a master's degree in health/physical education, and his doctorate is in curriculum studies. He used cultural studies as his framework for his doctoral dissertation, *The Oppression of Obesity*.

Dr. Johnson's doctoral research on weight bias was a phenomenological study, with cultural studies as the theoretical framework. This included the influence of media and corporations on weight bias, weight gain, and the targeting of overweight individuals as a consumer group.

Dr. Johnson has taught wellness/fitness at the collegiate level and has successfully provided fitness and life coaching to groups and individuals including children, general population, and athletes. Dr. Johnson recently contributed to the development of an International Diploma in Fitness and Scholastic Sports for the Malaysian Ministry of Education. Dr. Johnson is an international speaker in fitness and education who is represented by multiple speaking bureaus.

Mary Dimino is an actress, comedian, solo show writer and performer. She is author of the critically acclaimed stage play SCARED SKINNY: A one (hundred pound lighter) woman show, winner of the prestigious New York International Fringe Festival Overall Excellence Award for Outstanding Solo Show. After achieving and maintaining a weight loss of 115 pounds, "Mary exemplifies the hard work people do to lose pounds and stay healthy," as Meredith Vieira states. Weight is the defining battle of Mary's life and the heart of her comedy.

Mary Dimino is the winner of the 2010 MAC Award for Outstanding Female Comedian (Manhattan Association of Cabarets and Clubs). She is also a familiar face on television. You may have seen her luminous smile on NBC's Today Show, PBS, Comedy Central, VH-1, HBO's Chris Rock Show, New York Undercover, sketches on The Late Show with David Letterman, Late Night with Conan O'Brien, The Jon Stewart Show, American Movie Classics Network and in dozens of national commercials. She is a favorite studio warm-up for numerous New York based television series. In theaters, she plays Connie the Maid of Honor in the off-Broadway hit Tony and Tina's Wedding.

Mary is a contributing writer for various television shows, including the PBS documentary Fat: What No One is Telling You in which her personal journey towards health has been featured. The documentary follows Mary and others, giving viewers a window into the intense human dramas that rage inside people who have been labeled obese. It sheds insight into the complex human puzzle that is driving the obesity epidemic in America. For her work with PBS, she won a 2008 Gracie Allen Award, presented by American Woman in Radio & Television. The Gracie honors exemplary contributions of individuals who have encouraged the realistic and faceted portrayal of women in entertainment, commercials and featured programming.

Mary lives in New York with her husband and puppy.

Find out more about the authors at:
www.scared-skinny.com
www.encoreedutainment.com
www.marydimino.com
www.scaredskinnynomore.com

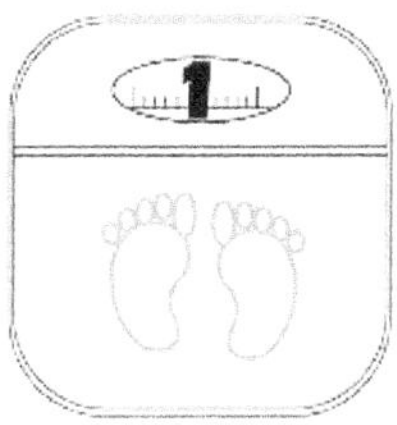

Fat: A Four-Letter Word

If you are like me, you wake up every morning, step on the scale and hope to see three numbers that will make your day.

Stepping on the scale is as automatic as drinking that first cup of coffee, taking a shower and feeding the hungry dog. Everyday we are weighing in. Why do we base our goals - even worse, our happiness - on this thing called *a scale*?

Much like Pavlov's good old dogs, conditioned to respond to the dinner bell, we too have been conditioned to respond to the scale. The number it reveals to us each morning will dictate our attitudes for the entire day. If it is lower than anticipated, we are ecstatic, with new leases on life. If the number is higher (even by one digit) – well, watch out world it's going to be a bad day.

I think of my goal weight all the time, that *ideal* number I'm supposed to weigh. I fear that I may never reach it. I hope that I will. I visualize the number. I dream about the number. I play Lotto with the number. I think I can. I think I can. I think I can... I am the little chubby girl that could.

I check in with the scale five, six times a day to see if I am getting any closer to realizing my desires (as if weighing myself repeatedly will help me lose ten pounds in a day). Hey, why not? Stranger things have happened. I once gained five pounds in an hour.

I put myself through grueling work out sessions, but the scale will not budge. It has a mind of its own. I must out smart it. I strategize. Tomorrow I will eat only water and tic tacs. The next day, I'll get a colon cleanse. A new hairstyle might shake things up. Yes, that's it! I will weigh myself after my haircut, starving, cleansed and naked.

Next time I better take off my jewelry - and my glasses.

After months of this (who am I fooling), years of this obsessive thinking, I've decided that I have had it. Yes, my friend, I snapped. I took the batteries out of my scale, hid it on the top shelf of a closet and smiled. NO MORE! No more will I be made to feel inferior by a number staring at me. I will live my life fearlessly, confident in the knowledge that I am happy and healthy.

I now realize that fear is not a just scale. Clarity - ah, clarity is the balance to weigh a life.

FAULT ZONES

We give the scale so much control over our lives. That's no surprise, considering exactly how much we have been conditioned to believe that we need to be skinny. Look at any magazine, movie or television program and that very perception is being reinforced. Yet ironically, research suggests that being underweight poses more health problems than being slightly overweight. So what's the deal?

Here's the deal. It's not all your fault. Yes, I've said it. It's not all your fault.

There is more than enough blame to go around, so stop placing it all on your own shoulders.

Of course there is always personal responsibility for all that we do, but there are many factors happening around you every day of which you are not aware. The food you're buying, the magazines you're reading, the family you live with, the restaurants in which you're dining, your favorite television shows you're watching; they are all making you fat!

This book will change your life. It will empower you and give you what you need to finally be healthy. Let's start with foundations within society's structure that affect our weight loss. That would be something called *weight bias*. What in the world is weight bias? Well simply, it is a societal attitude that makes you fat. It occurs when a culture insinuates that you have some defect, some abnormality if you are not thin. Then they bombard you with diet pills, dieting programs and quick weight loss gimmicks to help you become thin and thereby acceptable. Like loyal canines, we are conditioned to salivate at these promises. We respond by spending billions of dollars a year on weight loss products. After all, we have to be thin, we have to be normal, by gosh, we have to be accepted! And if we are unable to get as skinny as we should, we then buy into society's belief that we are undesirable, lazy and worthless. Yes, we've been manipulated into wanting to be painfully thin, and may I stress the word *painfully* here.

Believe me, I don't want to wallow in stories of victim hood for the sake of pity. No way Jose. What I do want you to know is that you are not alone, my dear friend, in this battle of the bulge. My goal is to educate you, help you make informed decisions, improve your health and improve the quality of your life. My wish for you is to never be manipulated into living a life in which you are constantly trying to live up to someone else's expectations or worse yet, to an unwitting society's unrealistic expectations.

Let's start by accepting the fact that weight bias exists in our culture. Objectively it is fact. Due to this fact, those who are overweight share many experiences and common characteristics. In this chapter, let's analyze weight bias, pick it apart, see what makes it tick. Let's hear from people who share the same exact experiences you may be going through right now. When we know better, we do better. Let's get you in the know.

Fat: The Final Frontier

Everything from technological advances, processed foods, media bias and the failure of fad diets has created a perfect storm scenario for weight obsession and oppression. Because there are so many factors that merged to create the obesity epidemic, most people don't understand how or what happened. Here are the factors that created this quagmire starting in the 1980's:

- Processed foods became a staple because of convenience and low cost.
- Exercise crazes increased the number of fad diets and diet products.
- Media exposure increased and skinny women became the industry standard.
- Advertising and corporations took advantage of processed food and the dieting explosion.

- Technology made life easier and more sedentary.

All these factors merged to ignite weight obsession and weight oppression within our culture. It is our very obsession with weight that has gone on to produce weight bias, an unfortunate side effect. Today fat is the last acceptable form of discrimination.

The Rise and Fall of Fat

Interestingly, before this confluence of events, excess weight was actually seen in a positive light. Being overweight meant that you were wealthy and had a higher status in society. In the 1800's, the snake oil salesmen sold weight gain elixirs to the public. Back then people were trying to put on the pounds almost as much as we are trying to take off the pounds today. From the eighties onward, the obsession with being skinny grew more intense. Even as late as the 1970's, the ideal woman was not a size 0 like Victoria Beckham or Jessica Alba but was a woman more like Marilyn Monroe, who happened to be a dress size 12. What a difference a decade (and some weight bias) makes.

Over the past three decades fat has become a four-letter word. If you are overweight, you are seen as lazy, unlovable and inferior to *normal* people. It is assumed to be Fatso's fault. Weight bias happens daily, inappropriately, painfully and abusively. Weight bias is not a statistic to those who experience it. It is not an epidemic, a disease. Weight bias is very real, very painful and very personal.

Gym Class Jitters

School was not a pleasant experience. The teasing was merciless. I couldn't fit into the latest brand name clothes everyone else was wearing, so I had to don what looked like tents more suited for Grandma from the Big Apple Circus. I know I can still recall, as you probably can as well for yourself, the many creative yet stinging names I was taunted with. I can still hear them in my head - Four Eyed Fatso, Chubb-E Chubs, Saggy Socks Sasquatch (yes, kids tend to like alliteration).

Because of society's stereotypes, bullying and name-calling are just the most observable byproducts. But the torture is even more insidious, remember, when no one wanted to sit by the fat kid at lunch, or told him that seat was saved for someone just because they didn't want him to sit there. My most hated memory of school was gym class. If there was a machine I could use to fast-forward me through time right to the end of that class, I would use it even if it meant messing up the entire space-time continuum. I despised everything about it; the choosing of teams, the locker rooms, the competing (my team's win or loss rests on my chubby little shoulders, what pressure!), the weighing in, the changing into the shorts and the teacher announcing your weight out loud. Oh, I'm starting to hyperventilate just thinking about it.

I always seemed to be one of the heaviest kids in class. I hated my body - was so ashamed of it, didn't want to run, didn't want any flab to jiggle, I barely wanted to move. I remember how much I wanted to play and at the same time had so much anxiety around the entire event that I was frozen by fear. Sometimes I'd even break out in a case of the jitters. I eventually begged for a doctor's note so that I could be excused from all physical education classes. Yes, I was the girl with the note, the girl that had something wrong with her, the girl who was too fat to run.

It is a tragedy that experiences like these happen to our children, to us. It's even sadder that they impact our lives in such a powerful way. And don't think for a moment that the teasing doesn't affect you throughout your life. Research shows that adults who were overweight as teenagers have an extremely negative body image and feelings of low self worth even as adults, even though the trauma happened decades ago. Sticks and stones may break my bones but words, well... words can hurt me for a long, long time.

The real pain for me started around age 12. That's when we become aware of our bodies, of our looks. We feel the pressure of society's expectations - to look good, to be like everyone else on television, in the music videos, in the magazines, to wear what the cool kids are wearing. We begin to mimic what we've heard our moms whisper to themselves, "I have to lose 10 pounds." "My arms look fat

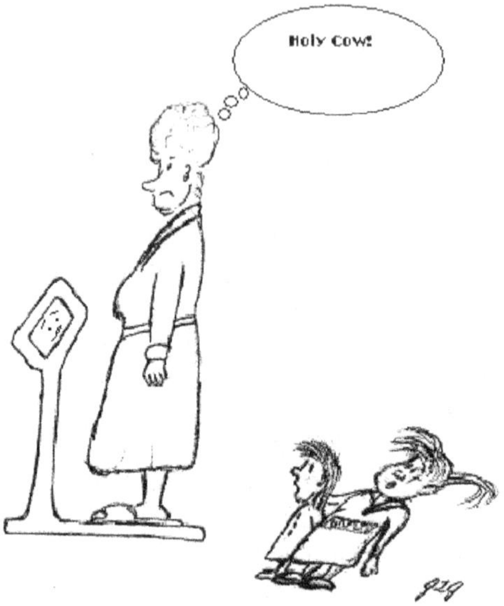

"Uh-oh, it's going to be a bad day!"

in sleeveless shirts." Or maybe the tried and true, "Do these pants make my ass look fat?" It all starts there.

An Inheritance

I have a childhood memory of my mother stepping onto our bathroom scale, looking up in disbelief, staring blankly into space as if her brain was plucked out of her skull and put into deep-freeze. Her lips mouthed, "Holy Cow, I can't believe I'm that fat..." as she drifted off into what seemed like a foreign dimension. The day went on and I could sense she was a bit aloof, somewhat preoccupied and simply not as happy as her usual lively self. To think that a scale and the number that was on it - whatever those three digits were, robbed her joy that day.

Like Grandma's fine china, that faithful day I inherited her outlook. What if I had witnessed something different? What if I saw a woman who was secure in her looks and her body? Would I have been even slightly different today? Would I be able to enjoy riding a bike outside not worrying if my cellulite is flopping around in the wind? How would I react to the scale today, when I step on it and see that it's not an ideal number? Would I shrug it off and go about my day in love with the fact that I am healthy and that I am a good person? Yes, just maybe, yes. Who knew that loving yourself really means loving your kids? The messages we give our daughters speak loudest in our actions, our words and our perceptions of our own bodies.

Insecurities are taught inadvertently, through the actions of our moms or even our siblings who may tease and make fun of our weight. In fact, about 30% of females report teasing from family, which leads to low self-esteem later in life. The way families treat each other reflects the attitude of our culture, the attitude that makes it acceptable to put down the overweight. We feel as though we have the moral high ground to make others so miserable that they will eventually want to lose weight. After all, they choose to be that way, no?

Obesity is the last acceptable form of discrimination. It is fine to tell someone they are fat but would you ever think of telling someone they are ugly as sin? "Here is a number, call it and get your nose fixed. You'll feel so much better." "Do something about that handicap, will you? How do you expect to ever get married like that?" You just don't hear people saying those things now, do you? However, you have probably heard insults such as, "Are you going to eat all that?" "Do you eat at buffets every meal?" Culture has empowered us to be biased against the overweight. And we inherited that bias. Ridiculing someone who is fat feels normal. In fact, it even makes you feel good about yourself. "At least I'm not *that* guy..."

Unrealistically Thin

Reinforcing our bias, the media bombards us with pictures of unrealistically thin people. I remember reading a teen magazine at age 14 about how to lose weight in a week. I was convinced I must lose weight. Why else would it be in writing, in a magazine? It must be true. And so the vicious cycle began - a cycle that took 20 years to finally break.

I can remember all the crazy fad diets and schemes I tried in order to lose weight.

From diet pills to cabbage soup dinners, to eating only bananas every day, to eating everything but bananas every day, to carb blockers, fat burners, ab rollers and cellulite creams. I could only imagine what I put my body through. The search for thin was so unhealthy. What were the end results? Simply this. Diets fail. Fads fade. Pills are dangerous. In the end, it is all about health, not a number on a scale.

Did you know? Approximately 1 out of 2 women are on a diet at any given moment

Love thy neighbor as thy self. How many times have we heard this and said, why yes, that sounds nice. But when it comes down to it, the sad truth is that some people really don't love themselves and they don't even know it. They find themselves having a hard time truly loving others, not knowing that it is within themselves that the love has to come from first.

Think about it, how difficult is it to love yourself when everyone is telling you that you are fat, unattractive, lazy, unmotivated - maybe even your own mother. Our culture has no redeeming value for obesity whatsoever. So why would you? Society allows weight to have such control over the value placed on self. It's either be skinny - or live in a world laden with ridicule, or worse yet, a world where you are invisible. Hey, everybody, can you see? There's a pink elephant in the room and it wants to go on a diet.

Do we actually believe that fat people don't think about their weight? Well, let me tell you something: they think about their weight nearly every waking moment of the day. Every time you need to move, walk up a flight of stairs, run for a bus, you are always aware of its presence. How could you not?

The Invisible Woman

When I was overweight, I'd swear I was invisible. I have been fortunate enough to lose 120 pounds, so I've experienced womanhood from each side of the scale. When

I was thin, doors were held open for me. Attentive male sales clerks helped me. I'd get smiles when I walked down the street. When I gained back 50 pounds that all stopped. Hold a door open? Yeah right. Help at the store? Just a shrug and a point. "If you don't see it, we don't have it," was all that was said, often without any eye contact. What a difference - being able to live this life from both sides of the spectrum of physicality. Ironic, but the larger a woman gets, the more disguised she becomes.

Overweight women experience greater bias associated with careers, relationships, friendships and socio-economic viability compared to their overweight male counterparts. Research shows that women who are overweight typically complete fewer years of school, are less likely to be married, have lower household incomes and have higher rates of household poverty.

Bias is experienced in every aspect of the lives of the obese; seats in stadiums, buses, airplanes and restaurants are not designed for the overweight. Therefore it makes it even more difficult for an overweight person to go out and really enjoy certain activities without feeling the shame that their weight carries. I remember watching one overweight lady boarding a ride at Six Flags. She was too large for the safety bar to close and everyone had to wait as they took her off the ride and walked her to the exit. I'm sure there were quiet remarks and jeers, but she didn't need them to be embarrassed. As her eyes welled up with tears, I knew at that moment she wished she truly were invisible.

I'm Not a Fat Cow; I Just Play One on TV

Celebrities and models are not immune from the pressures to be thin. In fact, some of them are scrutinized the most. Alison Sweeney recalls in her book how she battled her weight from her teenage years into her early twenties. She eventually was a dress size 12, not obese by medical standards, but still larger than her television peers. When she was starring in *Days of Our Lives*, she was 16 years old. She recalled getting a threatening letter from a viewer that read, "You FAT COW, leave Austin alone!" in big, angry letters. Incredible to believe someone even bothered putting a postage stamp on that. Sometimes the veil between reality and illusion can be quite thin, so to speak.

Even people that are overweight have been conditioned to hold a bias against people who are bigger than they are. As one plus sized model explains, "I still have people that won't work with me because they think I am too big for a shoot. When I am around the smaller models, I feel like they are judging me for my size. What's sad is that I feel that I do the very same thing to other women larger than me, like a size 20. I look at them and think they are too big."

Weight bias affects us personally, which in turn affects our relationships with others in society and even our own families. Culture plays a role in the discrimination. Unfortunately, when a woman achieves any level of success in our culture, her weight becomes even more of an issue. Is it any wonder that women often seek extreme dieting or develop eating disorders in order to maintain an unrealistic weight?

The cycle needs to be broken. It can start with you. There is a difference between concern and discrimination. When the latter is present, we need to voice our distaste and act towards understanding the true complexities that exist inside the life and body of an overweight person. This book will provide the strategies to help you understand what you can control and what you cannot, thus giving you the freedom to focus on what you can change. You will be scared skinny no more.

Weighing In

What have we learned? Weight bias is a part of our American culture and we continue to buy into it whole-heartedly, only for the lack of not knowing much else. We've delved into the abuse and oppression that the overweight encounter due to this ingrained bias. We've seen how our media influence us, taunt us and use our hopes to fulfill their economic agendas. There is so much blame to go around. There is no need for you to take all of it. Now that you know this, you can be empowered by it. Allow this newfound awareness to bolster you, give you strength to take personal responsibility towards health and wellness. Honestly, do you think anyone who is fat really wants to be fat? Did you ever hear anyone say, "If I could only be fatter I'd be so much happier"? Most people would do everything possible to be thin so they don't have to endure the pain and shame of weight bias. I want you to feel officially free, free of the pain weight bias has instilled in you. It is yours no longer.

Sometime during the reading of this book, you will "get it." I'm not sure exactly which sentence or which paragraph will be the one for you, but I do know that a light bulb will go off somewhere in your mind. You will get the secret knowledge needed in order to understand this thing called "fat." And that understanding will be the wind beneath your wings as you journey towards your road to total well-being. In all thy getting, my dear friend, get understanding.

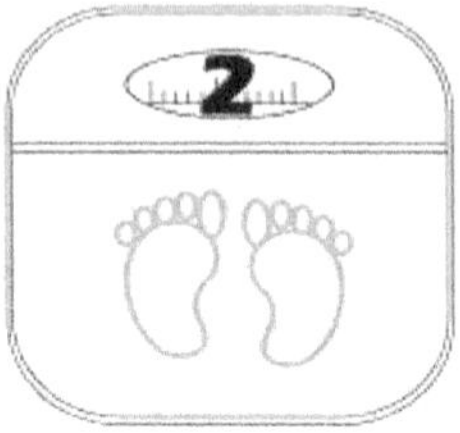

What You Don't Know is Making You Fat

Face it, as a nation we are getting fatter. There is no mistake about it. The question is why are we getting fatter? The typical person would say it is due to laziness. Get your fat bottom off the couch, put down the frosted donut hole and go to the gym. Wait a second, step back from the bias. If 66% of Americans are now obese, could that mean 66% of our country is lazy, unmotivated and just don't care? Could there be other factors causing obesity that we are not aware of?

Our eating habits have evolved from three meals prepared at home, to meals that are now eaten anywhere, any time. We practically have unlimited access to food. Beef jerky at a gas station, potato chips at the Laundromat. I envision a future with solar powered vending machines in the Mohave Dessert waiting to fulfill one's Double Stuff Oreo snacking habit while they are traipsing through the desert sands. Not only has the availability of food changed our eating habits, but technological advances have also changed our lives. As a culture, we are more sedentary. I can't remember the last time I got up to walk over to the television to change the channel. I think it was 1986, the year the Mets won the World Series. And today with laptops, iPods, gaming devices, universal remotes and Bluetooth, there is no need to ever leave the confines of your own couch. These are factors of obesity that we know, factors that are discernible. But what is it that we *don't* know that is making us fat?

Processed Food is Not Real Food

If you are under the age of 40, you probably can't remember life without processed foods. They began to flood the market in the late 70's and now make up most of the foods that are sold. It is impossible to walk down an aisle of a store without seeing a food product with an ingredient list that covers the entire side panel of the box. As opposed to actual food, like an orange for instance. What would that label read? Orange (grown on trees). Processed foods have become such a dominant part of our food industry that there are thousands of new products introduced each year. It has become a multi-billion-dollar industry. Businesses make their money by selling you products that are convenient, tasty (mainly from fats and sugar) and unfortunately enough, often geared toward children. Did you know that SpongeBob Macaroni is the bestselling macaroni product on the market? It's the same stuff; it just has SpongeBob on the front of the box. Kids see it and demand it.

The problem is this isn't really food but rather food "products," or simply faux foods. Call it what you like - phony bologna, sham ham or pseudo menudo; it is artificial food, and you've been eating it for decades. There is no Twinkie Tree, TV Dinner Farm, or a field where Cheese Doodles grow naturally in the wild. Processed foods have become such an integral part of our diet that we have long since forgotten that they aren't real foods. Interestingly, processed foods have been a staple in our diets since the epidemic rise in obesity began. Let's explore this phenomenon in more detail.

What are processed foods? Anything (and I stress *thing*) in a box, bag, can or package that has a shelf life of months or years. They usually have ingredient labels that look like a copy of the periodic table, cover half the package, and contain words that are tongue twisters to pronounce. As a farmer once put it, "If you can't grow it, milk it, or shoot it, well then you probably shouldn't eat it."

Faux foods are the predominant products now in grocery stores today. And 90% of all money spent by the consumer on food is spent on processed foods. We have it all upside down. What we should be spending: 90% of our grocery bill on fresh produce, fruit, vegetables and healthy meats, with only 10% being spent on boxed and canned goods.

Why are we fat? We are fat because we're eating fake food and we're feeding our children fake food. Why do we do this? Because that's what is available to us, that's what the food companies have developed for our consumption. To make matters worse, half of all meals are now consumed outside of the home (with 25% of those meals consisting of fast foods).

Our lifestyles have changed to a faster pace, so our dining habits have changed to accommodate our need for convenience. However, let's not cast blame on the Whopper or Big Mac simply because they exist. We, as a culture, have made processed foods the major source of our diet.

As a trusting culture, we assume that if the food is being sold, it is probably healthy enough for us to consume regularly. If it weren't good for us, then the food industry wouldn't be able to sell it. Let's look at this thought closely because it is blatantly incorrect. The food industry is interested in selling us food and selling us as much food as they can. They don't care whether we eat it, wear it, throw it away or hang it in a museum - they simply want us to buy more and more. But we wouldn't do that if it didn't taste so darn delicious. This is where the typical high fat and sugar contents come into play because, let's be honest, there isn't much that tastes better than fat and sugar. Except for fried fat and sugar. The food industry isn't interested in your health (that should be your job); they are interested in your money. This is not to say that the food industry is evil and conspiring to kill everyone off with obesity. If there were no consumers, they would go out of business. But I can say that the food industry does understand the types of food that our bodies like and so they focus on marketing that type of processed food for our consumption.

The accessibility of processed foods (particularly snacks) is due to one main ingredient, the god of all sweeteners, **HFCS (high fructose corn syrup)**. Scientists developed HFCS in the 1970's as a cheaper alternative to sugar. HFCS increases a product's shelf life, allows it to stay fresher longer and tastes really, really good. HFCS was a great boon to the food industry. It was an amazing discovery. Everyone loved it and found it a perfect fit for processed foods. HFCS is sweet, inexpensive and lasts long - everything a woman could want in a man...umm, I mean a sweetener. And the food industry latched on to its popularity. Today the average American consumes more than 62 pounds of HFCS per year. Scientific studies have shown that the rise of the use of HFCS in the United States mirrors the rapid rise in our culture's obesity. Yes, HFCS at first (like a bad boyfriend) seems so perfect on paper, but in reality he's a loser who lives in his mother's basement.

Another offender is **partially hydrogenated vegetable oil.** During the low fat craze of the 80's, butter and saturated fats became public enemy number one. So, partially hydrogenated vegetable oil was invented to make butter substitutes. "I can't believe it's not butter."

Well, it's not. It's a tub of trans fat! Trust me when I say, "I *can* believe it's not butter." These were put in many processed foods and can still be found in some today. There has been a push to remove trans fats from many foods, but that doesn't mean the foods are now healthy. For instance, Oreos no longer contain trans fats. However, it is still a processed cookie with all the other fats and sugars in there that make it so scrum delicious. The same thing with potato chips, the package prominently displays *no trans fats*, yet it is still a deep fried potato loaded with preservatives and chemicals. Which brings me to one scary point; we assume many of these processed foods are actually healthy for us.

I have learned to stay away from them. If it is food you buy at the drugstore or gas station, then it shouldn't be eaten. There is danger in the vending machines. The convenience of food should be a warning sign to us that we probably shouldn't eat it. Now we even have pink slime in ground beef and crushed cochineal beetles in your favorite strawberry-flavored Starbucks drinks. Yes, cochineal beetles are government approved for food, by the way.

Processed foods are not a healthy choice, no matter what the labels say. They are convenient and often cheap, which is what makes them so marketable. They are not foods that provide optimal health. To be healthy, you need to eat healthy foods, not fake foods. The body wasn't designed to process them.

There are 20,000 new food products being introduced each year, up from only 6,000 a few years ago. The Food and Drug Administration (FDA) maintains a list of over 3,000 chemicals that are added to the processed food supply. Some of these additives have never been tested for safety and require no government approval. Here are the top 10 reasons not to eat processed foods:

1. **Cancer** – Some cancers are caused by carcinogenic properties in processing of foods.
2. **Obesity** – Processed foods are most often high in fat, sugar and salt. If counting food calories, these are the main ingredients that cause excessive weight gain.
3. **High carbohydrates** – Most processed foods include an overabundance of carbohydrates and not nearly enough protein.
4. **Heart Disease** – The trans fat in many processed foods will spike the cholesterol level and lower the HDL.
5. **Hypertension** – Blood pressure is elevated by the high salt and fat content in these foods.
6. **Diabetes** – Foods high in sugar raises glucose to unhealthy levels.
7. **Additives** – For color, consistency, taste, shelf life and more, processed foods include additives while the effects remain unknown.
8. **Fillers** – Several foods like hot dogs and processed meats are filled with unknown parts.
9. **Empty calories** –Diets high in processed foods lack the nutrients needed to fight disease.
10. **Artificial vitamins** – Synthetic vitamins, which lose their potency during processing, are added to some processed foods, like bread for example.

There you have it; ten good reasons to eat real food, ten horrifying reasons not to eat fake food *products*.

Obesogens Abound

Have you ever heard of an Obesogen? No, it's not the new nickname kids at school are giving the chubby child. Nor is it the name of the pig on Green Acres. Obesogen is the term given to foreign chemical compounds that disrupt normal development and balance of lipid metabolism, which can lead to obesity. What exactly are they and where do they appear in our daily lives? They are chemicals that have been added to processed foods, plastics, pesticides and nonstick cookware. They are an unnecessary and mostly preventable hazard to our health. These chemicals are prevalent in our current culture and may have a large impact on how we gain and lose weight. Obesegens are making us obese.

Let's name the culprits:

Bisphenol-A (BPA) is an industrial chemical and organic compound that has been used in the production of plastics and resins such as the resin lining of tin cans, plastic food and beverage containers and even dental sealants. It is a synthetic estrogen that has been linked to ailments ranging from reproductive problems to heart disease, diabetes and obesity. Unfortunately, as in the case of canned tomatoes, acidity causes BPA to leak into your food. Researchers have studied bisphenol A's effects on estrogen function for more than a decade. Some scientists believe that developmental exposure to low doses of bisphenol A activates genetic mechanisms that promote fat-cell activity. In other words, it can make you fat.

High-fructose corn syrup (HFCS) is now classified as an obesogen. Acting on insulin and leptin in the body, HFCS potentially increases appetite and fat production. Basically, it makes you both hungrier and fatter.

Pesticides are substances used to prevent or destroy pests, and they have been used throughout history. Some pesticides persist for short periods of time and some for long periods of time, which are considered persistent organic pollutants (POPs). Several studies have shown pesticides as obesogens, linking them to obesity and diabetes. Americans are exposed to approximately 13 different pesticides through food, beverages and drinking water every day. And nine of the ten most common pesticides are endocrine disrupting, which have been linked to weight gain.

Pharmaceutical drugs are also potential obesogens. From 2005-2008, 11% of Americans aged 12 and over took **antidepressant medications**. Research suggests that certain antidepressants, known as selectively serotonin reuptake inhibitors (SSRIs), are potentially adding to obesity levels in the USA. One of the main functions of SSRI antidepressants is to regulate serotonin re-uptake transporter (SERT), which can affect food intake and lipid accumulation. This in turn can lead to obesity.

Organotins such as tributyltin (TBT) and triphenyltin (TPT) are tin-based chemicals. They are endocrine disruptors that have been shown to increase triglyceride storage in adipocytes. Common sources of human exposure include contaminated seafood and shellfish, fungicides on crops, anti-fungal agents used in wood treatments, industrial water systems and textiles. Organotins are also being used in the manufacture of PVC plastics and have been identified in drinking water and in the leaching from plastics.

Perfluorooctanoic acid (PFOA) is a surfactant used for reduction of friction and it is also used in nonstick cookware. PFOA's are used in food products such as the lining of microwave popcorn bags. In animal testing, the chemicals cause liver, testicular and pancreatic cancer. Studies show that microwaving causes the chemicals to vaporize and migrate into your popcorn. Researchers worry that levels in humans could approach the amounts causing cancers in laboratory animals. DuPont and other manufacturers have promised to phase out PFOA by 2015 under a voluntary EPA plan, but millions of bags of popcorn will be sold between now and then. PFOA has been detected in the blood of more than 98% of the general US population. Animal studies have shown that prenatal exposure to PFOA is linked to obesity when reaching adulthood.

Many more obesegens will be identified in the next few years. It is clear that these chemicals have an environmental impact on obesity. However, these products may cause more problems than simple weight gain, so it would be beneficial for us to rethink using everyday items containing these chemicals. Obesegens are hazardous to your health - and your waist.

Addicted to Food (Products)

"Over consumption of palatable food (chemically altered junk food) triggers addiction-like neuroadaptive responses in brain reward circuits." Nature Neuroscience 13, 635–641

Food products are highly addictive. One of the major struggles when it comes to controlling weight is food addiction. I know many people who have attended Over Eaters Anonymous because of a food addiction. It is so interesting that people who are addicted to smoking, gambling, alcohol, drugs and sex are given much more empathy than an over eater. Not many people think that food can be an addiction. We even tend to view other addictions as almost glamorous. Think of the attention a celebrity gets for going to drug rehab. Yet, many in society say that we can't be addicted to food. Whether the addiction is physical or emotional really doesn't change the fact that food can be addictive. What do I mean by addictive? Have you ever had a really bad day? What did you do when you got home? Did you take out a stalk of celery and eat it? No, you probably grabbed a bag of M&M's or the roll of cookie dough or the half-gallon of ice cream and shoveled the food in until you got your comfort fix. You feel better for a few minutes, maybe even a half an hour. Then the guilt kicks into high gear and you ask yourself, what just happened? Well, what happened was you got high, just like an addict.

Not everyone responds to food in this manner. There are people who don't like to eat when they are stressed. Then there are people, like yours truly, who desperately seek food when stressed. So what causes some of us to be addicted to food? We yearn for the carbohydrates because carbs help us with our serotonin levels. Serotonin is a chemical in the body that regulates your mood, or in other words, it makes you feel good. So when you consume carbohydrates it actually affects the body's ability to produce serotonin. The more you eat, the more serotonin is produced and the better you feel. However, when the mood elevation subsides, you will likely feel worse than you did before. This occurs partially because your insulin will spike leaving you feeling tired and partially because you will be depressed about the extra calories you have just eaten. As your tolerance for this high increases, your need for more carbohydrates to feel good also increases. It becomes a vicious cycle of overeating carbohydrates or reaching for them any time you are stressed.

Do you recall Spurlock from the documentary Super Size Me? He was a fit guy that decided to eat fast food for a month. He got sick when he first ate it because his body was not used to consuming processed foods. But, over the course of the documentary, we see a man literally become addicted to fast food. At one point he is feeling physically bad, but when he orders the food, he gets excited, almost childlike in his exuberance of getting to eat it. He has become addicted to the processed food high. However, after the meal his blood sugar spikes and then quickly drops and he is sitting there in an almost catatonic state.

Many people share this addiction to food. For some it may be emotional eating, for others eating out of boredom, and for some it might be a physical craving related to carbohydrates. Regardless, the effect is the same. The food makes us feel good so it becomes a drug of choice. I know the first thing I'd do after a long, stressful day is reach for both the comfort food and the remote. It has become routine. It was an automatic response to the stress of the day. Some of my favorite comfort foods, which are usually high in carbohydrates, were potato chips, ice cream and buttered bread. If this sounds familiar, you may be a carbohydrate junkie. Become cognizant of your addictions so that you can change your habits. Learn to enjoy coming home and unwinding in a different way. Working out is a fabulous option that sounds difficult at first, but for me I know that once I'm 15 minutes in, I'm golden.

Food addiction can be a physical or an emotional issue. The physical addiction can be broken by eating simple, natural foods. The emotional addiction can be helped by becoming more fully aware of what you are eating and why. Ask yourself; do I really need this right now? What am I feeling while I eat this? Is there anything else I can be doing to help me relax? Questioning with awareness is the first step in breaking an addiction to food.

Limit the amount of processed foods you purchase at the grocery store and at fast food restaurants. When shopping, read the labels and see what foods are packed with fats, sugars and chemicals that are addictive to the body. Use common sense in your purchasing choices. Have you ever heard of anyone addicted to salad, or who reaches for a carrot when they are feeling depressed? No, because these aren't foods that increase serotonin in the brain and give you the same high that you can get from junk food. Temper temptation by staying away from triggering faux foods.

Technology Created a Sedentary Culture

We are all hopped up on the fake food and then what do we do? We sit. And we sit, and we sit. A sedentary lifestyle does not mean that people are getting lazier, but rather technological advances, less active leisurely pursuits and increased sedentary jobs all contribute to a culture that is less active than in the past. Could we ever live without these advances? Not me. I love my remote control. With that one piece of plastic, I can turn on the television, surround sound, DVD player, satellite dish and even close the garage door.

However, a sedentary lifestyle should be expected because the American dream is to make life as convenient and easy as possible. So in effect, we are more sedentary because of the success of our culture. Even our phones have one button speed dial so that we don't have to press the whole ten digits. When was the last time you washed a sink full of dishes rather than put them in the dishwasher? Doesn't seem like that big of a deal until you realize all of the advances really do make our lives more inactive.

As early as the 1980's, it was evident that obesity was likely to increase through the rise in technology. Just a couple of decades ago, many jobs were physical in nature, but today most jobs are sedentary. With the decrease in physically demanding jobs, most adults do not compensate by engaging in regular exercise.

What else has changed? Our lifestyles. Children today come home and spend endless hours playing video games, watching television or surfing the net. When I was a child I was constantly outdoors with friends, swinging on swings in the playground. If I came indoors, my mom would make me go back outside until dinner was ready. It's not just our children who've had changes in lifestyles, but adults too. How often do you come home from work exhausted or stressed, you don't have the energy to do something productive, so you spread out on the sofa and watch Dancing with the Stars. I find that ironic. Instead of actually getting out and dancing (which would give us more energy and relieve stress) we are sitting watching other people dance.

And usually we do this while eating Doritos and an array of other processed faux food snacks. We've traded comfort and decompression time for mental acuity and health.

Television. Who doesn't love that brilliant invention by Marconi? I can't get enough of it. That wonderful mega screen idiot box now has 1.7 million channels compared to only 4 channels just three decades ago. We even place our furniture strategically around the television. We spend our lives in the living room, around it - barely living. (Feng Shui provided by Sony and RCA.) Rooms are dedicated to the large screened siren calling us to come and sit and watch. Today most of us own more than one TV. We claim they are all necessary, yet my great grandparents never even owned one and they survived. Heck, even thrived. They had conversations in the evenings with each other. Amazing huh, families actually talking to each other about their day.

For many people, television has become their lives. Today there is a cable station for anything that may peak your interest. There is a wedding channel, wealth channel, comedy channel, food channel, even a channel to help you familiarize yourself with all the other channels. The average viewing time per day has risen from 2 hours in the 1970's to 5 hours per day in the 1990's.

I am now going to blow your mind. Read this at your own peril. This has changed my life. Here goes. There was a study that discovered people burn fewer calories while watching television than they do at rest! Yes, you burn more calories staring at the wall than watching the wide screen that's hanging *on* the wall. Television viewing not only makes your metabolism slow down, it also slows down the mind! The boob tube will make your butt larger and you dumber. What a lethal combination.

Technology has changed our lifestyles from 30 years ago. Today we spend hours surfing the internet, playing games online, looking at screens all day. One of the most important changes that can be made in our families' daily lives is to limit the amount of screen time. This is not to say that technological advances are bad. What person would want to wash their clothes on a rock at the creek, or talk on a phone with a chord tethered to the base unit in the kitchen? Technology is really kind of cool. Our advancements catapult us into new areas of possibility. And nothing is cooler than that. But we need to use technology smartly, to serve us, not to work against us. Ultimately, we need to assess our leisure time and make changes that are more physically active to compensate for our newfound sedentary lifestyles.

Stress Influences Weight

You would think with all that sitting, fast eating, and convenient life-styling, life would be a walk in the park - or maybe a sit on a folding chair in the park. But that's not so. From the moment the alarm clock buzzes until we fall exhausted into the bed, we deal with stress. We have pressures dealing with money, family, friends, careers, traffic and a dozen other stressors that fill our lives every day.

Having stress isn't necessarily a bad thing. The commute is bad, but you have a job. You hate the mortgage payment, but you have a home. You just had an argument with your spouse or sibling, but you have someone in your life that cares about you. Stress can take a toll on our bodies and it is how we deal with stress that can affect our weight and our health.

Imagine, if you will, the stress associated with obesity. Think of all the biases you may endure each day. The limited job market, dating, social life, and even your doctor thinks you are lazy. To make things worse, you are dieting (or more likely starving), buying every low fat food on the market, and developing a sports injury just trying to walk around the neighborhood. Most overweight and obese individuals feel they have little control over their lives.

What areas of life do you have control over? The food you eat is one of the major sources of control. Because of this control, eating to ease stress can be a physical and even mental addiction. But what is noteworthy is that how the body reacts to food (whether eaten due to an addiction or eaten due to stress) is very similar. When we reach for fattening comfort foods during stressful times, it may be an attempt to self-medicate, to raise our serotonin levels in order to feel better. It gives us immediate relief from the stresses of life. Not surprisingly, people under stress don't tend to make smart food choices.

A chemical in the body that affects weight is **cortisol**. Researchers have discovered that chronic stress causes the body to release excess cortisol, a hormone critical in managing fat storage and energy use in the human body. Cortisol is known to increase appetite and may encourage cravings for sugary or fatty foods. Increased cortisol levels also influences the storage of body fat, particularly "visceral" abdominal body fat. **Visceral fat** is stored deeper in the abdominal cavity and around the internal organs. This visceral belly fat is particularly unhealthy because it is a risk factor for heart disease and diabetes. In other words, stress goes right to your belly!

More recent studies also suggest that our bodies may process food differently when we're under stress. Research studies performed on mice and monkeys fed a diet high in fat and sugar gained significant amounts of body fat when placed under stressful conditions. The animals fed a normal diet however, didn't gain as much weight despite stress. Researchers linked that phenomenon to a molecule called **neuropeptide Y** (NPY) that is released from nerve cells during stress and encourages fat accumulation. A diet high in fat and sugar appears to further promote the release of NPY. This also causes a build up of fat in the abdominal region (visceral fat), which is considered the unhealthiest deposits of fat in the body.

This type of visceral fat storage affects everyone, even skinny people. Yes, someone who looks skinny may actually have large amounts of fat deposited around organs, especially if they are not active. And it appears that stress can influence this as well. One of the ways to deal with stress is to understand it and be proactive in preventing it when possible. Here are a few tips that will serve you well and keep the visceral tummy fat at bay. I like to call them my stress busters (rather than gut busters, which more likely involve reaching for cake). So if you're a recently unemployed parapsychologist who catches ghosts on your free time, or just the average person catching the hassles of modern day life, you should call on these tips also. Who you gonna call? Stress Busters! I ain't afraid of no stress.

Stress Busters:

- Get up fifteen minutes earlier in the morning. Starting late or feeling rushed increases stress throughout the day.
- Prepare for the morning the evening before. Set the breakfast table, make lunches and put out the clothes you plan to wear.
- If you have a job that requires a lot of sitting, stretch and walk around occasionally.
- Get adequate sleep. Going to bed earlier is more beneficial than sleeping late.
- Focus on positives, not negatives. (Be glad you have the job, not focusing on the long commute.)
- Make time for yourself (meditation, spa, yoga, time with friends)
- Talk it out. Discuss your problems with a trusted friend or loved one.

- Eat healthy foods. Even snacks should be healthy choices.
- Remember that most of the things we worry about don't actual happen. And if they do, it's usually not to the extent that you worried about.
- Remain ever thankful and focus on the positives in your life. At the end of the day, it's not your job or car that will keep you going, it is family, friends and love. Have an attitude of gratitude.

We all have certain amounts of stress in our lives. And those of us who aren't skinny deal with more than our fair share. Much like dealing with your problems, you can sit around and do nothing or you can make a decision to change your habits. Become proactive to stress rather than simply reacting to it. Being proactive means removing the junk food from the cupboard and replacing it with healthy choices, in case you do have a bad day and need some comfort food. The only thing worse than binging on junk food after a bad day is the guilt of eating the junk food after a bad day. This guilt causes you to eat even more or increases your stress at the very least. Being reactive is a vicious cycle that we need to step out of. "Last stop, Guilt-Ville. Stand clear of the closing doors please." It's time to get off the crazy train of reactive thinking that leads us to a destination we know all too well.

Weighing In

Yes, what you don't know can make you fat. Culture affects weight gain. It is absurd to believe 66% of the population is overweight merely because they choose to be, especially when you consider all the negative associations with obesity. Technology is a great thing, but it has made us a less active society. And, as you will learn in future chapters, your body was designed to move.

Obesogens are making us fat - and sick. Obesogens are what we should be scared of rather than if we are skinny enough for society's liking. If they are as harmful as research suggests, then we each need to make an effort to remove them from our daily lives. Take what you've learned here and put it to use simply by being aware of it. But don't freak out. This doesn't mean you can never eat a fast food burger again or can never buy your favorite processed snack cake. What it means is that you now know these foods aren't the best choice for optimal health. Use them sparingly, as opposed to the hyper consumption in which you are being programmed for by corporate advertising. Now you know what is making you fat. When you know more, you do more. And you do better.

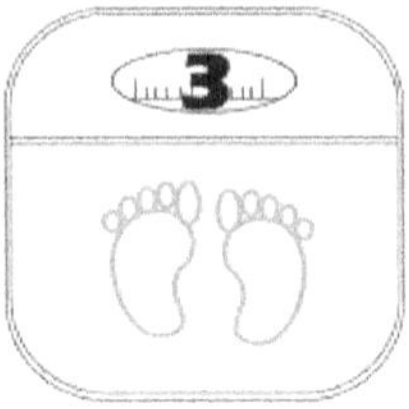

Mass Media Manipulation

Technology has created an empire. The media, television, advertising and news outlets now have the power to influence like never before. Since the media embrace the vision of fat being repulsive, they have perpetuated the biases associated with obesity and provide venues for the diet industry to target overweight people.

Even though the consensus is that obesity is evil, this consensus is not founded in science. Instead government has manipulated the media. They've also been manipulated by the movie industry and even by experts with a nefarious agenda.

Interestingly, advertisers will fill the airwaves with fast food commercials, but when you eat their food and gain weight, it is your fault. So advertisers then fill the airwaves with commercials for weight loss products to make you acceptable (skinny) again. The media portrays skinny people as fun, healthy, beautiful and admired. The consensus that skinny is beautiful has been manipulated by the media and corporations since the 1980's.

We are assaulted with marketing genius that targets popular foods, tasty foods and foods that well, just make us fat. You may have just finished eating lunch, you walk outside and see a 40-foot billboard for a sundae, and so you desire to eat a sundae. Think of those catchy jingles like *you deserve a break today.* How cool is that little ditty? I always tend to agree with it. Why, yes, I do deserve a break today. When I stop lying on this couch, I'm going to take a well-deserved break and head for McDonald's. While there, I'll pick up a Happy Meal for the kids. It will make them very happy. Hmm, I wonder how many Happy Meals they would sell if they called it a Crappy Meal?

Advertisers Spend Billions So You Overeat

The weight epidemic involves a paradox, a corporate paradox. What do I mean? Corporations are a major reason for America's weight gain. They create faux foods and then spend millions on advertising to get you to want them. Advertising is geared toward selling large quantities of food to consumers. These foods have little to do with nutrition, but rather with a large profit margin.

For instance, the Corn Growers Association is spending millions of dollars on an ad to convince the public that HFCS (high fructose corn syrup) is actually a natural and healthy ingredient in foods, an ingredient that actually makes food better. But have you ever seen the corn industry make a commercial promoting the consumption of, oh I don't know, corn? No, you haven't. And you never will because corn doesn't have a large enough profit margin to justify spending millions on advertising. Yet HFCS does. It is a staple in most processed foods and could cost them potentially hundreds of millions of dollars if people stopped consuming foods with HFCS. It is incredibly bombastic that they are trying to convince us that HFCS is actually healthy and derived from a natural source. Is a laboratory really a natural source? Plus they are trying to compare it to natural sugar as a reason to consume it. But in reality sugar needs to be consumed sparingly. So, either way you look at it, their logic is flawed.

Consider how faux food has become a part of our daily lives. All thanks to creative marketing and the money that greases the industry's wheels. Let's look at statistics: By 1998, 89% of children under the age of eight had visited a McDonald's at least once a month (the Vice President of marketing said his goal was to make it 100% by 1999). McDonald's is not the only fast food company that has experienced phenomenal growth over the past two decades. However, they have excelled in brand recognition, which serves them well in dominating the fast food business. Studies show that the Golden Arches are more recognizable around the world than the Christian cross. And Ronald McDonald is the second most recognized fictional character on earth—second only to Santa Claus. Now that's advertising at its best. To think, the two most recognized characters in the world are a fat guy in a red suit and some clown.

Advertising has become a major influence in our culture as well. In one study, researchers examined the taste preferences of young children (3-5 years old) based upon the influence of branding from a heavily marketed source. The children sampled identical foods that were either in McDonald's packaging or in plain packaging. The results of the taste test revealed the following:

- Seventy-seven percent of the kids said the same French fries from McDonald's were better in a McDonald's bag than in a plain bag (13% liked the ones in the plain bag; 10% could tell they were the same).
- Fifty-four percent of the kids said carrots tasted better in a McDonald's bag (23% liked them in a plain bag; another 23% could tell they were the same).
- Sixty-one percent of the kids said milk tasted better in a McDonald's cup (21% liked milk in a plain cup; 18% could tell it was the same).
- Fifty-nine percent of the kids said chicken nuggets tasted better in a McDonald's bag (18% liked them in a plain bag; 23% could tell they were the same).

Here's an idea; in order to get kids to eat their vegetables, just put them in a McDonald's wrapper. Genius, I tell you!

Another study examined how advertising is targeting our children. This study found only 10 nutrition related advertisements compared to 564 food advertisements during 52 hours of Saturday morning television viewing. The vast majority of these advertisements were for fast foods, soft drinks, sugary snacks and candy, which are the opposite of healthy food sources that are recommended for growing children (Kotz, & Story, 1994). The problem with commercials geared towards children is that children can't differentiate between commercials and programming and therefore don't understand the intent to sell products. Seventy percent of children ages six through eight believe fast food is healthier than food prepared at home, largely because of commercials.

Another powerful strategy of major corporations has been to partner with television and movie companies to flood the market with brand name foods. Over 30 billion dollars a year is spent on branding - food boxes graced with characters from Beauty and the Beast, Toy Story, Sponge Bob, Blue's Clues and other irresistible cartoon favorites. Children love the cartoon and so assume the food product must be great, too. Most of the products linked to television or movie characters are typically processed foods that are high in fat, sugar and calories. Even the fast food industries have used this concept to ensure high consumption, as in the case of McDonald's and Burger King often including Disney characters with their children's meals.

Corporations have exorbitant budgets when it comes to advertising because it works. Successful ad campaigns dramatically increase sales. McDonald's *you deserve a break today* campaign bolstered sales from 587 million dollars in 1970 to nearly 2 billion dollars in just 4 years. We've become conditioned by corporations to buy their products because they make us feel like we need them. How many times have you been watching television late at night and a thick, juicy hamburger flashes onto the screen. You hear it calling your name. You may even seriously contemplate going to eat it right then. Even if you don't, it pops up in your mind again for lunch the next day and you find yourself pulling up to the drive-thru window asking for the number 2 special, super-sized.

These corporations don't spend billions on advertising for you to eat there once a month. They want you to eat there every meal. So they offer toys to children, discounted prices to parents and super-sized meals for the hungry. Once or twice a month is enough when it comes to eating fast food. Try to wait until it is necessary, such as when you don't have time to fix dinner because you're taking the kids to Karate class. Remember - balance is key, Grasshopper.

Weight Loss Foods Scare You Into Buying Them

If you're overweight you may not feel good about yourself, and in those dark hours, when seeing yourself as a monster, any advertising offering a way out will seem like the answer. The industry creates commercials that make the consumer feel inadequate. Without their great product, you'll remain a loser.

And really, who wants to be a loser? None of us. We take part in our own reality series Scared Skinny every day. Similar to *Fear Factor*, we compete in alarming exercises in futility, force ourselves to eat disgusting food, swallow pills with side-effects yet unknown, inundate our senses with advertisements warning us of our weight, all in order to win a prize. And the prize is SKINNY - or elimination, which in real life is death, whichever comes first. And who is the winner? The weight loss industry because it is worth $55 billion in the US alone.

We are targeted as consumers, which is worse than just being a focus of ridicule because they use our guilt and shame to make money off of us. We are walking targets with bullseyes on our backs, bellies and butts awaiting the impact of skinny's arrow. Our culture has established thinness as the standard for health, beauty and even morality. Advertisements for weight loss pills and programs such as Jenny Craig or Weight Watchers target the overweight with the message that they have a defect that can only be cured by buying their product. This focus on weight loss has not gone unnoticed by the food industry either. Today there are literally hundreds of processed foods that are made to be low fat, low-carb, low calorie, light or even "diet" to cater to an ever increasing number of dieters looking for a solution to their weight loss needs. Since most Americans view obesity as an individual moral failure, rather than the result of processed foods and environmental factors, obese individuals are often willing to try any method to help.

Society's obsession with weight has created a market for specialized products, such as diet foods that are targeted toward the overweight, with the intent of making you buy the product to make you a healthier person. Corporations target the insecurities of consumers, but especially those as vulnerable as the obese. As long as we allow the stereotype to exist that people are overweight because it's their choice, the advertising industry will continue to target and exploit this vulnerable group.

The Blame Game

Corporate America is perpetuating the rise in obesity, then blaming the consumer for their obesity, and then offering solutions to overcome obesity, only to once again blame the consumer when the solutions are ineffective. A corporate paradox. Since we are so confused about what works, what doesn't work, who is being truthful and who is not, you can see how we are motivated by fear and frozen in the headlights just waiting like sitting ducks.

Think of how advertising is geared toward women. For instance, there is a supplement called SlimQuick on the market that is targeted specifically at women. The commercial shows a dieting cartoon female that loses weight only in her boobs. It then shows the same woman on SlimQuick and she loses all the weight in her stomach and hips while her boobs remain the same, if not bigger! Now that's targeting, on more than one level.

There is a product called Akavar that actually claims it will make you lose weight without dieting or exercise. It states, "We couldn't say it on TV if it wasn't true." So thousands of people spend their hard earned money only to find out that, yes Virginia, you can say it on TV, even if it's not true.

One interviewee shared, "I would have to say that I think most diet companies and weight loss pills target everyone. Most of the pills, equipment and meals are meant to make those who are only slightly overweight feel like they need those products to take off the last few pounds. And even more so for people who need to lose 20-30 pounds, which kind of encompasses everyone."

Always remind yourself that the weight loss business is a multi-billion dollar industry with a 95% failure rate. If you think about it rationally, you'll realize that if any one of the products were effective, then all the other products would be obsolete. Can you think of any other product that you would consider purchasing if it had a guaranteed failure rate of 95%? Yet, every year thousands of new weight loss products arrive on the market waiting for a sucker - I mean a consumer, to purchase them.

Advertising works and it is especially effective for weight loss. The $55 billion Americans spend on weight loss products annually is equal to the Gross Domestic Product (GDP) of the Dominican Republic. The only thing getting bigger than us from dieting is the bank accounts of the weight loss companies who prey on dieters and then blame them for their failure. Keep in mind, if it sounds too good to be true then it is. No pill is going to help you lose 10 pounds of fat in a week. So don't get caught up in the fear of weight. Your goal is to be healthy and still have money in your pocket. Eating right and becoming more active doesn't require you to take out a second mortgage on your home in order to afford your new health.

The Media Perpetuates a Greater Bias Against Women

Women endure the greatest public bias because of their weight. This may be due to a male dominated culture creating a mindset that women should be thin and beautiful and that men who are overweight can still be strong and powerful. The media idealizes women who are skinny, so whoever doesn't fit into that mold is seen as undesirable. Regardless of the achievements a woman attains, she is ultimately measured by her waist size and not her wallet size. Ironically, the more successful a woman becomes, the greater the scrutiny of her size.

Isn't the media just reflecting what's already out there? Or do we merely imitate what we see in the media? Well, both. Let's start with the latter. There is no doubt that we are influenced by what we see. In grammar school, I saw Dorothy Hamill's haircut and next thing you know, all the kids in school, including me, were asking for a Dorothy Hamill at Super Cuts. Sure, we are influenced by what we see. In fact, over the last 20 years, the number of skinny women in the media has increased from 38% to 76%. That means currently only 23% of the women we see every day in television and magazines represent the average (or above) weight!

In the media men encounter less bias than women. Fat men are a little more acceptable. On TV for instance, Jackie Gleason, John Candy, Chris Farley, John Belushi, the classic comedians were often overweight and were acceptable. Today's counterparts Kevin James, Jack Black are not just acceptable, they are considered sexy. Then there are older guys that have gained weight like John Travolta, but they are still accepted and not targeted like their female counterparts. You will not hear that Tom Hanks gained another 5 pounds in the news or see pictures of him at a heavier weight on the beach, plastered all over tabloid covers at the checkout line.

But people like Oprah, Roseanne, Kirstie Alley and Lindsay Hollister are always under scrutiny by the media. When they gain a few pounds it is talked about. Overweight females in entertainment programming are usually seen as evil, sad or even tragic characters. Remember Mimi on the Drew Carey Show when they put makeup on her like a clown and made her an evil character. Or do you recall 'Fat Monica' on *Friends*, lonely and eating donuts? In fact, I can't think of one Disney princess who isn't thin and beautiful, but you can be sure that their evil step-mothers and archrivals are usually gravitationally challenged.

Many roles for heavy people, especially women, may have actresses only a few pounds overweight trying out for the role. Today producers think that a size 10 is large. A size zero seems to be the trend, wasting women away to where they don't even look like women anymore. I remember after Patricia Arquette was pregnant and she still carried some extra weight from her pregnancy, the media were ruthless in attacking her. She was outraged when she was asked to lose her baby weight for her role as psychic detective Allison Dubois in the TV series *Medium* – because the character is a mother of three. Outrageous, she just had a child and was now told to lose weight so she can look like a character would who have three children. Her response to the producer when asked to lose weight was, "I don't want to do this job then because, to be honest with you, I'm trying to make little changes in the world. If it made any sense for this part – if this part was a supermodel or anorexic – then okay. But DuBois is a mother of three in a long-term marriage. It doesn't make sense." Thank you, Patricia, for standing up for yourself, for us all.

Women endure the greatest bias for being overweight—both in the media and in American society. Unfortunately, this appears to empower or justify the attacks on women who are overweight. The media stereotypes fat women. Sure, overweight men in the media still endure stereotypes and bias but not to the extent that women endure. For example, look at the unfair bias expressed in shows such as *King of Queens* or *Still Standing*, where overweight men are married to thin, beautiful women. How many shows have we seen where a fat woman would be married to a thin, handsome man?

Thin and beautiful at all costs, ladies. That's the message we get every day from our television, movies and magazines. We feel bad about ourselves when we open Vogue and see models that look like they haven't eaten a hot meal in weeks. How can I ever look as glamorous as her? Well, that weight-loss ad on page 172 might help! Maybe not eating breakfast and lunch today, that'll do it. Sure, I can starve 10 pounds off my body this week for that high school reunion. It's making me skinny, yes, but is it making me healthy? No. It is just reinforcing the idea that you need to be uncomfortable to be thin and beautiful.

What about men? What advertisements are targeted toward them? There are a few weight loss programs that have men as spokespeople now, such as Terry Bradshaw for Nutrisystem, but these types of advertisements are not common. What are common ads for men? They are targeted with ads to get bigger and stronger with sports supplements. Or perhaps a truck ad. Rather than the new and improved weight loss pill targeted for women, men get targeted for the new and improved beer. Who knows, maybe a guy can get big and strong enough to bench-press a couple of skinny models, that would possibly make him "the most interesting man in the world."

Results Not Typical

Don't you just love the commercials where someone looks so down-trodden in the before picture and suddenly, in the after picture they are shining with joy, lots of make-up and a new hair-do to boot. And then, all the way at the bottom, in small, tiny, itsy bitsy print, barely perceptible to the human eye, there's the disclaimer, RESULTS NOT TYPICAL. Isn't that a kick in the head? Getting across the message that if you are not skinny, you are defective and we can help. But if we can't, don't blame us, fat ass! (And by the way, results not typical.) We have been conditioned to believe that if the product we've purchased doesn't work, it must be our fault. By gosh, the people in the commercial are getting great results all the time. What's that you say? I didn't hear you. The paid actors' results in the commercial usually don't happen for people who use the actual product? Now you tell me? Typical...

Weighing In

The media is schizophrenic in their behavior regarding obesity. One minute there is a commercial selling ice cream and the very next minute there is a commercial showing an overweight woman eating ice cream - but the latter is for a weight loss pill. And people wonder why our culture also acts schizophrenic about weight loss.

Unfortunately, this insanity is now pressuring the next generation to be thin or be outcast as well. Media bias has a profound effect upon the body image of adolescents, especially females. Research concludes that magazines have a strong influence on girls' perception of their weight and size. Sixty-nine percent stated that magazine pictures influence their idea of the perfect body shape, and 47% reported wanting to lose weight because of magazine pictures. There's also a correlation between the frequency of reading women's magazines and the prevalence of having dieted to lose weight. These studies illustrate that the media perpetuates weight bias and influences one's perception of self, even if that perception is based upon unrealistic images. Incredibly, even girls in 5th grade already feel pressure to be skinny. It's not like school isn't hard enough, now a girl has to worry if her butt looks big in her desk?

If you can change your attitude about the whole weight epidemic, imagine how much pressure will be taken off of our daughters, nieces and granddaughters of upcoming generations. Let's not depend upon the government, media or anyone else to take control of our lives. Let's take back the reins. If you really want to empower this generation and generations to come, understand that the media manipulates us happily, it's just what they do. And what you can do is be aware of it. The time is now to take back control of our lives.

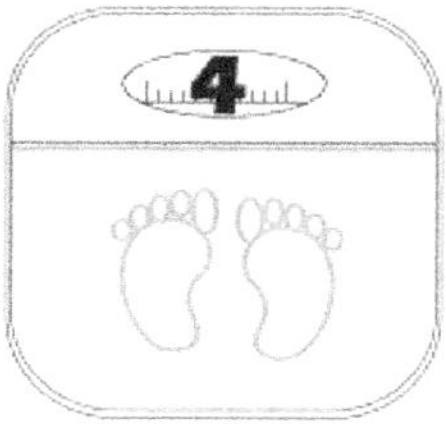

Fad Diets are for Skinny Bitches

Once upon a time two former models (who've been blessed with never having to lose any weight) wrote a book telling us how to lose weight. They called it *Skinny Bitch.* It was publicized as "a no-nonsense, tough-love guide for savvy girls who want to stop eating crap and start looking fabulous." I guess some of us girls are just not savvy enough to look as fabulous as them, unless we become skinny bitches, that is. These ectomorphs don't know any more about weight loss than they would about how to gain muscle mass or how not to be born fabulous. Unfortunately, because of the pressures of "tough-love" from the fabulously skinny, most of us are willing to try even the most ridiculous fad diets and listen to the most inappropriate people for their advice.

At any given moment half of all women are on a diet. If you are like me, it's probably not your first diet either. Much like waking up every morning and getting on the scale, going on a diet is a lifestyle for some of us. Why do we endlessly attempt dozens of different diets? Because diets don't work, that's why! It is a fact that 95% of dieters gain back all the weight lost, and then some.

As the title of this chapter suggests, diets can work for skinny people and herein lays the problem. Fad diets work for a short period of time for a certain type of person, who only needs to lose a few pounds. Who are these people? They are typically young skinny women in the movie or fashion industry.

Let's face it; diets have been around forever, probably since Eve ate that first apple and felt guilty about it. But fad diets increased in popularity during the 1980's to levels never before seen. The increase in technology, an exercise craze, increase in media exposure, and a change in the cultural view of weight all collided to create the stage for fad dieting. There are now well over 100 different fad diets that consist of everything from the lemon diet to the cabbage soup diet and every skinny bitch diet in between.

A seismic shift in culture and technology created an environment where fat is now seen as nothing short of evil. It was this shift, brought on by a multitude of factors that made weight one of the main focuses in the late 20th and 21st Century. So, the media turned to celebrities to see what they were doing to keep the weight off. Unfortunately for us, most celebrities are different than the general population; otherwise they would be part of the general public rather than celebrities.

Many celebs are somewhere between a size 0 and size 2 or 4. So, when they go on a diet, it is to lose only a few pounds in a short period of time. Yet, when they lose weight it is publicized on television, magazines and in articles all over the internet. They are the people that the media seeks due to their fame. These diets then become fads for everyone to try so that they can also look like a Megan Fox, Cameron Diaz or some other actress.

The problem with these fad diets is that most women are not a 25 year old actress that has never had a child and is genetically a skinny body type. If these people were really overweight or had less active lives, then the fad diets would not work for them either.

Dieting Makes You Fatter

It is statistically proven that dieters will gain back all of the weight lost and probably even more within 1 to 5 years. All that hard work to wind up weighing more than before you started? What's amazing about psychology is that even though something doesn't work, we keep trying. In fact, that is the definition of insanity: to do the same thing over and over expecting a different outcome. We are always searching for the one diet that will change our lives. Why? We fear being fat. We fear the weight bias that comes with being fat.

Although dieting has a near perfect failure rate, people still take extreme measures to lose weight, which include succumbing to eating disorders, self-starvation, surgeries and even the use of prescription pills. Why is there an apparent Scared Skinny epidemic in our culture? As stated in previous chapters, the last accepted discrimination is obesity. We are motivated by revulsion because it is the one discrimination that everyone has the potential to endure. Regardless of your race, age, or socioeconomic level - anyone can gain weight. It is the one common prejudice that anyone can experience.

We are willing to try anything to stave off the oppression of being overweight. If standing on your head while singing the theme song to Shaft guaranteed weight loss, then that would surely be the next fad. And there are programs out there just as inane, and people still flock to them. There is nothing in the world that has evoked as much fear, hatred and bias than the thought of being fat.

Diets don't work long term because our bodies are designed based upon the feast or famine concept. When there is restricted food intake such as when dieting, the body reacts by going into famine mode. The body slows down its metabolism and actually burns calories at a slower rate than when it is getting adequate food. The other problem is that the body also tries to hold onto fat as much as possible if it thinks food is not readily available. So, when someone significantly restricts food intake the body will actually try to breakdown and use muscle tissue for energy and hold on to the fat. When you diet your body does all that it can to retain its fat! In fact, if you diet without exercise, as much as 40% of weight loss can be muscle. Dieting can actually make us lose muscle, make our breasts smaller and increase the size of our thighs and buttocks.

Have you ever watched *The Biggest Loser*? This show is designed to see who can lose the most weight over a period of time. Everyone thought it was the answer to weight loss because most of the contestants lost a lot of weight. The contestants left the show with the intention of keeping the weight off forever. Now fast-forward nearly a decade from when the show first aired in 2004. It may or may not surprise you to know that many of the contestants have gained most of their weight back. Season one winner Ryan Benson regained all of his 122 pounds lost on the show. He admitted in interviews that he'd starve himself and lived on "cleansing beverages" in the weeks leading up to the finale. Immediately after the show he gained 30 pounds just by hydrating. In 2008, he starred in the indie film *DISfigured* about a few friends in a fat acceptance group. Ryan was cast as "an overweight man." Imagine all that work, fame and even reward only to return to the size he was before. Dieting is a vicious cycle.

Today it has become fashionable to be on the latest diet. How many conversations with your friends focus on which diets you are on? Some of today's diets may be minutely successful for the short term, but this is because you are actually paying attention to what you eat, or more likely, what you are not eating. The point is you are focusing on your diet, which makes some success possible, but does not mean that the diets themselves are what you'd want to follow for a lifetime. For example, you could simply not eat for a few days and lose weight, but here again this is not healthy and does not build a foundation for long-term success with weight management and improved health. Health is a process, a state of awareness (which is what this book is now heightening in you) that involves many facets of your life, not just what you eat or don't eat.

The other problem with most diets is that one nutrient is typically removed from the diet. This is where the low-carbohydrate and low-fat diets come into play. When one nutrient is lacking, our bodies actually begin to crave it. If you are thirsty, don't you drink water to quench the thirst? Well, if your body is void of carbohydrates for example, your body will thirst for them as well. We have been programmed to think if we eat any carbohydrates on a low-carb diet that we are failures. When in reality the body needs them. Once carbohydrates are reintroduced to the diet, weight gain is almost guaranteed because any excess will be stored as body fat.

Comedian John Pinette discusses his experiences with low-carb dieting. He said he was told that he would crave carbohydrates but after a few weeks the cravings would subside. He said, "I felt lied to.... a couple of weeks later I was driving by a Krispy Kreme and jumped out of a moving car... now that's a craving." How many of us have felt that way too? When we deprive the body of needed nutrients it is going to crave them. By not eating what our body needs to live just because we want to lose weight, is like someone not seeing the forest for the trees - or more appropriately, missing the donut by looking through the hole.

Finally, consider the experience of one friend who explains that when she turned 30 she was so fed up with dieting that she went to an obesity center, which she said was like a grown up fat camp. She spent a month (and $10,000) to lose only 2 pounds. A month of being diligent, measuring food and exercising hard got her nowhere. It cost her $5,000 per pound. She could've spent that money on a month long trip to Hawaii and probably would have lost two pounds just by swimming in Maui and enjoying the wonderful food. Like a bolt of lightning, Wendy said that she had an epiphany when she stood on that scale at the end of that month. She decided she was done with trying to look a certain way. Stick a fork in it, done. Not done caring, but done allowing dieting to control her life.

Maybe the following experience of a friend of mine sounds familiar to you. Every Monday she would sit down for lunch and have the latest fad diet scheme ready to turn her 270-pound body into a 120-pound model by Friday. By Tuesday she'd get discouraged because she wasn't successful, decide the diet wasn't right for her and would then eat a fast food burger with fries. While eating the hamburger she'd tell me about a new diet she just heard of and would start next Monday. She'd definitely be more dedicated to that one. And she was, till Wednesday or Thursday.

Low Fat Food Makes You Fat

I was one of those people you see with a shopping cart full of low fat cakes, low fat cookies, low fat everything that is available. I was taught that it was good to buy everything low fat. I wasn't told that most low fat food is riddled with sugar and processed HFCS instead. For example, a

Snackwell Cookies Sandwich Crème Packs 2 Go has 210 calories per serving with 38 grams of carbohydrates and 18 grams of sugar. Hey Snackwell, is this really snacking well?

It's about as healthy as a tub of lard. But because they are marketed as healthy, we not only buy them but also eat more of them. How many times have you eaten a whole box of low fat cookies because they were, after all, low fat? However, low fat foods aren't necessarily low calorie and they certainly aren't low sugar. Low fat diets actually made us fat. The experts didn't tell us that. Think of all the excess carbohydrates that have been consumed because of the low fat craze touted by so many.

When low fat dieting only made us fatter, the "experts" then decided we needed a low-carb diet. But as you've learned, the low-carbohydrate diet doesn't work either. Because once you start consuming back carbohydrates, you are going to blow up like a puffer fish. Some of the other fad diets include the Grapefruit Diet, the Mailbu Beach Diet, the Stop the Insanity Diet (which seems very fitting, by the way). Eventually we just give up and return to our old friend, the See Food Diet.

As mentioned earlier about female athletes, when is the last time you saw one of them living on low fat cookies or low carbohydrate brownies? More than likely you never have because they know these foods are not part of a healthy diet.

There are also diet foods that claim to make you healthy. However, they are highly processed, highly unhealthy and are a major factor in our weight gain. Rather than reach for real food, we turn to diet foods so laden with artificial ingredients that our livers work overtime to process them.

Did you know the packaged foods of diet programs such as Weight Watchers, Jenny Craig and Nutrisystem are full of chemicals and processed ingredients much like other regular processed foods. Here is the ingredient panel of Macaroni and cheese from Nutrisystem:

ENRICHED MACARONI (DURUM SEMOLINA FLOUR (WHEAT), NIACIN, FERROUS SULFATE, THIAMINE MONONITRATE, RIBOFLAVIN, FOLIC ACID), CHEESE POWDER (MILK, CHEESE CULTURE, SALT, ENZYME), MODIFIED CORN STARCH, INULIN, WHEY PROTEIN CONCENTRATE, NATURAL FLAVORS (CHEESE, YEAST EXTRACT, SODIUM CASEINATE, MONO AND DIGLYCERIDES, GUM ARABIC), ONION POWDER, TETRASODIUM PYROPHOSPHATE, BUTTERMILK POWDER, SOUR CREAM POWDER, DISODIUM PHOSPHATE, POTASSIUM CHLORIDE, GARLIC POWDER, DEXTROSE, XANTHAN GUM, LACTIC ACID, SOYBEAN OIL, LACTOSE, MALTODEXTRIN, CITRIC ACID, NATURAL TOCOPHEROLS, ANNATTO POWDER, FD&C YELLOW #5, SILICON DIOXIDE. CONTAINS MILK AND WHEAT

Is this something we should eat or something we should clean our toilet with? It looks like a list of answers to a chemistry exam. The only real difference between these foods and other processed foods are the prices. A serving of macaroni from one of these programs has approximately 200 calories and may cost around $4.50. However, Kraft Easy Mac Macaroni & Cheese has 220 calories per serving and only cost about $1.00 per serving. While neither one is the healthiest choice, why would you spend more money for basically the same product?

The only other difference between normally processed foods and diet foods is that they add less fat or an artificial sweetener is added to reduce calories. These foods could probably sit on a shelf for a year or more and not spoil. They are as well preserved, if not more, than government protected Wetlands. Some of these foods don't even need refrigeration. There is actually chicken salad that doesn't need to ever go in a refrigerator! To me that's not chicken, that's trick-en - chicken's evil imposter. If it sounds like chicken and it looks like chicken but lasts longer on the shelf than paint thinner, it's probably not chicken.

Diet program companies aren't the only ones selling these products. Most food suppliers realize that there is a large market for diet foods. However, if you have ever tried these food products you realize that there may be something not right about them. For example, there are products on the market such as low carb ice cream, which is supposed to be okay to eat if you're a low carb dieter. I bought a half-gallon once and it tasted so bad I left the ice cream in my kitchen sink. I woke up the next morning and found a big glob of gelatinous goop. To my horror, last night's ice cream never melted! That's how well preserved it was. That's how non-ice cream it was. I scream, you scream, we all scream for faux ice cream.

Do you know how hard it is for the body to digest that? Do we even know the long term effects stuff like that can have on our organs? But even the foods we think as normal diet fare, like Lean Cuisine, Smart Ones and Healthy Choice are all highly processed products that are full of preservatives and ingredients that are not really a healthy choice after all.

You have probably heard the old saying *caveat emptor* or *let the buyer beware*. Well, I say *caveat titulus* or simply, *beware of the label.* If a food has to tell you it's healthy on the packaging, then you might want to ask yourself why. I have never seen a sticker on an apple that read *health food.* I saw an advertisement for hot pockets the other day. Now any intelligent human being knows that a hot pocket is about as healthy as smoking a menthol cigarette, yet the commercial actually tried to persuade me that since the hot pocket contained real cheese and had no trans fats that it was a healthy food choice. And this wasn't even one of their lean hot pockets no less. Yet think of all the hot pockets they will sell by saying that in their advertisement. And think of all the gelatinous goop that your liver will need to clean away, if it even can.

I am not trying to single out any food company or any particular food product. The point here is to make you aware of the fact that these are not healthy choices. Could you imagine your great grandmother reading this label? She would probably think it was for a product that cleans kitchen cabinets. Today in our society, we suck down these ingredients like they are as natural and nutritious as carrots. And yet we wonder why there is such an increase in obesity, diabetes and cancer in our culture.

The Not-So-Magical Magic Pill

The market is flooded with thousands of products that make outrageous claims such as *Lose 10 pounds in one week* or *Lose 30 pounds in 30 days.* Some of them target women by promising to make them lose weight in only "all the right areas." These types of promises include anything from prescription pills, to health food supplements, to obnoxious drinks that are guaranteed to make you skinny (and vomit if you don't hold your nose when swallowing it).

There have been actresses that have tried weight loss pills. Unfortunately, they also have access to prescription drugs such as **amphetamines** or even illegal drugs such as **clenbuterol** to lose weight. These diet products can usually help you lose weight but that's because they are loaded with caffeine, ephedrine or some other metabolic stimulating ingredients. Prescription weight loss pills typically contain ingredients such as **Phentermine, Sibutramine,** and **Orlistat.**

These products speed up your metabolism, suppress appetite or may even prevent fat from being absorbed from food. When you discontinue using the pill and your metabolism returns to normal, you unintentionally gain it all back. The diet pills that suppress appetite run great risks such as dizziness, heart palpitations and tremors.

Taking diet pills for weight loss is similar to taking Tylenol for a headache. You don't have a headache because your body is deficient in Tylenol. The Tylenol simply treats a symptom but the root cause is still there. It is the same with these pills. Your body isn't lacking ephedrine or phentermine - they simply treat a symptom rather than the root cause. This is why there is no long-term success with these products just like with fad dieting.

I admit I am guilty of trying some of these diet pills. While they may have had short-term success, the lasting effects for me could have been severely harmful and even fatal. As one interviewee shared of her experiences with diet pills, "I tried every over the counter diet pill, I tried Fen Phen, Meridia and I tried a $400 a month diet supplement to help me lose weight. I even did the Zone Gourmet, which was $1400 a month. I tried everything to lose the weight. But now looking back, I wonder what the effect that drugs like Fen Phen had on my metabolism and body. I wonder if it actually caused me to gain weight after I stopped taking it."

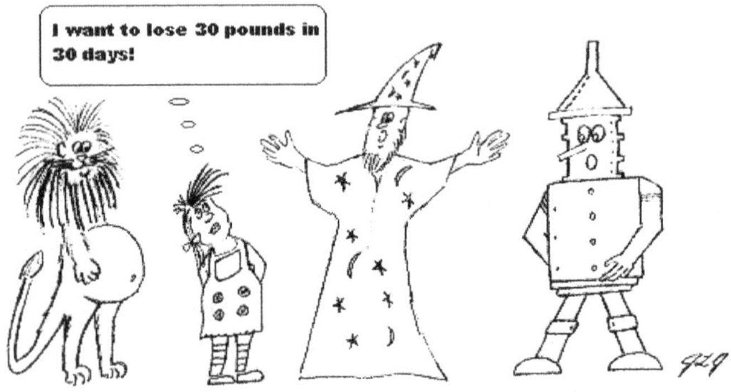

"I'm afraid I'll need a more realistic timetable."

Does she sound anything like you or someone close to you? Most women who have struggled with weight will tell you that they have tried nearly every diet pill on the market and usually wind up weighing more after surviving the horrendous experience. We get caught in its cycle. A diet fails, we think it is our fault because we couldn't commit to it enough; we become depressed and choose to diet again. Similar to the lion in The Wizard of Oz who believes his problem is lack of courage, we believe our problem is lack of commitment.

Our founding fathers risked their lives for liberty and the pursuit of freedom. Today we are risking our lives for the pursuit of thinness. In fact, prescription drugs may pose even greater risk to your health than over the counter pills. Some of these drugs have been determined to cause major health problems and be potentially deadly. **Fen-Phen** is one such drug that was shown to cause heart valve abnormalities. The FDA removed it from the market. Due to similar safety concerns, Sibutramine was also removed from the US market by its manufacturer.

Another increasingly popular method of dieting is weight loss centers, where medical experts are supposed to help you lose weight. These are different than the typical weight loss programs like Weight Watchers. These medical weight loss centers claim to be comprised of physicians who have specialized training and expertise in the field of weight loss. But how effective are they? These centers typically prescribe over the counter weight loss pills as part of their weight loss programs!

Pills are not the answer. Here is a list of some of the typical ingredients in OTC (over the counter) and prescription weight loss pills:

(OTC) over the counter weight loss pills	**Prescription weight loss pills**
Stimulants: Ephedrine (derived from Ma Huang, Yohimbe) Caffeine (derived from Kola Nut, Guarana, Green tea) **Appetite suppressants:** Hoodia Gordonii Glucomannan (soluble fiber) Garcinia cambogia	**Stimulants:** Amphetamines Phentermine Phenylpropanolamine Sibutramine **Appetite suppressants:** Phentermine Phendimetrazine Diethylpropion

The side effects and dangers of diet pills can vary because many contain a blend of ingredients and the dosage instructions vary from product to product. However, possible side effects include: nervousness, dizziness, headache, back pain, constipation, nausea, anxiety, insomnia, diarrhea, blurred vision, elevated heart rate, palpitations, elevated blood pressure, heart failure and even death. Sexy, right? Who doesn't love a thin, beautiful woman with bowel issues? Better yet, I can just get really thin and die. This way everyone will remember me as being skinny forever.

Many companies have been fined by the FDA or sued by consumers because of misrepresentation in the health claims of their products. The FDA has banned certain ingredients like ephedrine at different times due to potential health risks. Taking these supplements is a crapshoot, where the reward definitely doesn't outweigh the risk. Even if you don't incur these side effects, your body will react when you stop taking the supplements.

Your metabolism will be so out of whack that you will probably gain back the weight fairly rapidly. *Take at your own risk.*

Pathological Dieting is an Eating Disorder

When we hear the words eating disorder, we may think of anorexia and bulimia. However dieting along with the frequent and compulsive weighing that accompanies it, can lead to eating disorders. According to one source, people who diet are eight times as likely to develop an eating disorder as people who don't.

Dieting is like a gateway drug into a world where we always need our fix. Studies show that 35% of "normal dieters" progress to pathological dieting. Of those, 25% progress to partial or full-syndrome eating disorders. Approximately 10 million women and one million men in the United States struggle with anorexia and bulimia. There are another 25 million who suffer from binge-eating disorder. There is an epidemic of eating disorders in our country that is causing more serious effects than being overweight.

Women who are thin feel the pressure to be even thinner. We often look at the women in Hollywood with disgust because they are a size 4, 2, or even 0. But, they feel the same pressure as everyone else. In fact, they may feel it more because of the unrealistic expectations of women in movies and television to be stick thin. These women are also constantly dieting, much like us who are larger. However, they often go to more extreme measures so they can land that next role and maintain their star status in the public eye.

One actress shared her story of dealing with the pressures of Hollywood. The weight loss started before she went to LA because she knew she would need to be thin to get work. When she started booking jobs, it pushed her to diet harder because she thought the work was coming in because she was smaller. She said because there is no security or control in the industry, controlling her eating habits and weight was her one source of power and control. She developed anorexia. Even though she wasn't eating much at all, food was her obsession. She thought about it all the time. In fact, she didn't think she was anorexic because she thought about food so much. She remembered that previously she had weighed 120 pounds, but now she was worried she weighed too much. When she stepped on the scale now, she weighed only 100 pounds. She felt good about the number she saw, but in her mind she felt like her body was still was too big.

Sadly, this isn't an isolated case, but in fact this could have been one of a hundred actresses in Hollywood who share very similar experiences. When I hear this, it makes me pause and rethink my sorrow for these women who feel the need to be so thin. They in fact face the same bias and pressures that we do in larger bodies. My empathy and sadness becomes tinged with anger when I think that if a 100 pound actress can still feel fat, then what chance would a regular woman ever have in learning to accept her body? Sometimes the outlook seems bleak.

This is my question to you. When you are on a diet, are you really focused on a healthy diet? Are you only focused on the weight loss? Be honest. If the answer is no, you are not focused on a healthy diet, then you are probably balancing on the verge of an eating disorder. The two are really closer than you might think. Here are some interesting points taken from a holistic-based residential behavioral health treatment facility. For our purposes, when you see eating disorder, I'd like you to replace it with fad diet.

- A healthy diet is focused on healthy weight loss. An eating disorder (fad diet) is an unhealthy way to lose weight.
- A healthy diet makes your body stronger. An eating disorder (fad diet) makes the body weaker and can cause numerous health complications.
- A healthy diet can be enjoyable and still allows one to live life. An eating disorder (fad diet) is not enjoyable and takes over a person's life.
- A healthy diet requires that you eat varied foods in moderation. An eating disorder (fad diet) often causes a person to eat very large or very small portions of a limited amount of foods.

- A healthy diet is about helping yourself become healthier and stronger. An eating disorder (fad diet) focuses on what others think of you and draws attention for the wrong reasons.
- A healthy diet affects one's health and choice of foods. An eating disorder (fad diet) affects every aspect of life.

It is evident that most of the dieting that occurs in our culture is more closely aligned to eating disorders than it is to a healthy form of dieting. This alone should completely change your view about the harm of dieting. The harm is not just physical, which is bad enough, but it is mental and emotional as well. If you are honest with yourself, you may realize that you have allowed dieting to take control of your life. Do you wake up every day ready to deny yourself food because you think you aren't skinny enough? Does it control your every waking thought? When is the last time you ate a piece of food and you didn't feel guilty about it?

Another issue related to dieting for women deals with control. Often women feel like controlling the amount of food they eat is the only real control they have in their lives. When the diets do not work, which they never do long term, women feel more self doubt and defeat. This is a vicious cycle, which leads to more extreme dieting methods.

What about the health risks of dieting? Sudden death from heart arrhythmia or electrolyte imbalance is a real risk. Each year dieting is related to severe health damage and deaths in the United States. Dieting focuses attention on appearance, rather than self-worth, health and personal fulfillment. Dieting mothers become role models for dieting children. It's time to break this deadly cycle.

Weighing In

The fitness craze along with increased media scrutiny created a culture of bias toward fat. This perfect storm created a destructive path that has left millions of overweight women in its path. Unfortunately, fad diets seemed like a quick fix to the weight problem. That is why there have been literally hundreds of them developed since the 1980's. Eating disorders often developed because of this fad dieting.

As fad diets ultimately failed, diet foods and diet pills were created to continue the pursuit for the perfect body. Even the perfect body changed from the size 12 of Marilyn Monroe of the 1950's and 1960's to the size 0 of a Kate Hudson today.

Diet food programs can be very expensive. The total costs of these various programs and their food products can be as much as $800 to $1,000 per month. This is for one person. I know 300-pound football players who don't spend anywhere near that much money on food per month, and those guys can eat. Yes, it takes a little work to buy natural foods and prepare them, but isn't your body and your health worth only the best?

Once you get into a routine of eating less food products out of boxes and packages, your tastes buds will begin to appreciate the beautiful flavors of real food as opposed to the techno-colored flavors of fake.

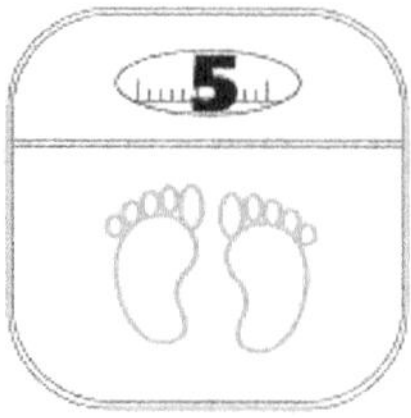

Real Women Have Butts

Is there an ideal weight? Is thinner really healthier? The answers will surprise you. There are so many myths, lies and deceptions associated with the answers. I am here to expose them. Let's start by learning that the human body is comprised of three different *body types*: ectomorphic, mesomorphic and endomorphic. These three basic body type combinations are what make us all come in different shapes and sizes - and there is nothing anyone can do to change that fact. Real women have butts.

Though we may differ greatly in life, we are all created equal. Humanity shares a wonderful gene that ultimately seeks truth and freedom. Sure, women may be more communicative and empathetic. But a few good guy friends will help you on moving day. We each have our strengths within the unity of our equality. However, there is one place where women and men differ greatly, and that's *body shape*. Even though men and women both come in varying shapes, men seem to be more accepting of their body types than women. When it really comes down to it, you can't change your genetics. If you are four foot nine, you will always be four foot nine. Unless, of course, you are wearing stiletto heels or you're strapped onto a Medieval stretching rack, which are basically similar tortures in my opinion.

Why do we find it so hard to accept our body shape? If you got curves, good! Let's dress those curves so they complement you. Shop for clothes according to *your* figure, not the model's figure in the magazine. We can look ravishing if we only shopped according to our bodies, be it pear, apple or any luscious fruit you may be. It's all good because under that body, there is *you*. And you come from a long line of fabulous genetics.

Embrace your shape. Embrace what makes you different. No matter how much I've always wanted to be Brooke Shields, I grew up to be me. No surgery can add 8 inches to my height. No workout can change my hip structure. One buttock cheek cannot be removed, even if I have one that is big enough for both of them. I can safely say that my butt will never qualify to be Brazilian. I need to embrace my uniqueness, along with my flaws and what I think are my weaknesses. The very thing you hate about yourself is the one thing that may endear you to someone else. We all want what another person has. And there is someone else that wants what you have! I have a friend with no butt at all. She's always complaining that her pants never look good, and would pay anything to have my big ole butt. It's an interesting mantra, but I've come to learn that the key to success is to want what you have. From there, positive transformations occur. The planet would be a dull and useless place if everyone on it were the same. Find your perfection in your imperfections. Celebrate what makes us all different, rather than judge each other because of those differences.

Why do women seem to have no problem torturing themselves with diets and surgeries in the hopes of achieving a body acceptable to society? It is a fact that most men are not attracted to unrealistically thin women. Men like women of all shapes and sizes who are healthy and most of all, confident. We need to do the work for ourselves, not for anyone else - not to impress a man, a woman, a competitive friend. For our unique selves we must do the work, so that we can harness our power and lead fulfilling lives.

There is No Ideal Weight

A common theme in dieting, and in this book for that matter, is the ominous bathroom scale. We look to it for validation. We have been conditioned to think there is an ideal number that will make our lives perfect. However, there is no ideal weight. In fact, one of the methods that have manipulated us for decades is the height-weight tables. You know, the ones that say what you should weigh based upon your height. The acceptable range is termed to be *desirable* or *ideal.* Desirable? What does this mean? Desirable to whom?

Weight-charts are yet another instance where if you don't fall within a narrow scope of what is considered desirable or acceptable, then you are obviously undesirable or unacceptable. A concept of an ideal weight leads to further weight bias.

Height-weight tables have been around well over one hundred years. Around the turn of the century, life insurance companies began to use them as a means to determine life insurance costs. In 1943, the Metropolitan Life Insurance Company introduced their standard height-weight tables for men and women. The tables were revised slightly in 1983. They were written as *desirable weights*, and would indicate those persons with the lowest mortality rates. However, the phrase *ideal weight* gradually became associated with these tables in common usage, even though the word ideal was not specifically published with the tables. What was the purpose of these tables? They were created to help the insurance companies make a profit. If people didn't fit into ideal weight categories, then they could charge them higher premiums or deny them insurance altogether. This meant larger profits for the insurance companies. It was all about money, not health.

Unfortunately, there is little research to validate the height-weight charts. Dr. Steven Blair, an obesity expert at the University of South Carolina states, "If the height-weight charts say you are 5 pounds too heavy, or even 50 pounds or more too heavy, it is of little or no consequence health-wise, as long as you are physically fit. On the other hand, if you are a couch potato, being thin provides absolutely no assurance of good health and does nothing to increase your chances of living a long life."

Height-weight ratio does not indicate the health of an individual. Arnold Schwarzenegger, who is in the Guinness Book of World Records as the fittest man in the world, would have been considered obese at the time, according to these height-weight tables. This is completely absurd. It makes you wonder how so many of these myths become so entrenched into our culture. Even within the height-weight tables they have added frame sizes so that now there is another variable in the mix. This only reinforces the fact that there really is not an ideal body weight. In fact, if you are eating healthy and exercising, you may actually be gaining muscle, which would increase your weight. This would make you even more overweight on this type of table, but in reality your overall health and fitness level would be improving.

There are many more flaws with the height-weight tables, such as not accounting for different body types or body shapes. However, the biggest flaw is that it doesn't account for body composition. Body composition is the ratio of lean body mass to body fat. Look at an athlete like tennis pro Serena Williams. She is 5'9" and weighs about 170 pounds. This would be considered right on the line between overweight and obese. Yet you can see her abdominal muscles. If someone has a six-pack for abs, they are clearly not overweight.

Have you ever stepped on one of those height-weight scales at a public store and it then asks you to enter your height, age and sex? Unfortunately, there isn't a *none of your business* button on any of them. After putting in the 50 cents or dollar, it asks for your information and then takes, what seems like an eternity, to weigh you. You wait on a slip of paper that not only tells you how fat you are, but the ideal weight you *should* be. And this ideal weight always seems to be closer to a slab of brisket, or possibly your body minus head and arms.

We read that piece of paper and depression sinks us faster than the Titanic, all because we have fed into the belief that there really is an ideal weight for us. Our focus should not be on a chart or a number on a scale, it should be on health - and healthy doesn't know an exact pound. If you cannot be active with your family or enjoy life to the fullest, then it is time to make healthy lifestyle changes. However, pursuing an ideal weight is not healthy, it is an enigma.

You Can't Change Your Body Type

There are tall women, short women, large women and small women. There are women that are big boned and there are women with very thin, almost fragile looking bodies. If you have a Kathy Bates body shape, you will not look like Kate Moss. It doesn't matter how much you eat or don't eat, there are certain limits that you will be able to achieve based upon your body type and genetics. Most of the fashion models you see in magazines typically are young women and haven't had children yet. Once they've had children, they will probably look very different. So if you are 30 or older, have children and are 5'2, there is a very real possibility that you will never ever look like Jessica Alba. The goal should be to look ***your*** best, not to look someone else's best.

Women place a great deal of self worth on their body image. Millions are spent on advertising targeted at women to get them to want products that will make them "look and feel better." However, for the average American woman the reality is that she will never have the body, features or height of a super model. Even if one did manage to get that ultra thin celebrity body, think what one needs to go through to get it. You can start by simply not eating, and then move on to developing a life threatening eating disorder. Next, there is the chic Hollywood thing to do, hire a personal chef and a personal trainer. Unless you are very wealthy, that's probably not an option. Besides all that, there is one fact remaining - the majority of women just don't have the body type to be ultra thin.

Women look towards the media for examples of what they should look like. But what women need to know is that many of the females we see in media are ectomorphs (small-framed body types). Not too often do you see a short, large-framed woman starring in television or film, even if she isn't "fat." In fact, being fat or obese is technically subjective and quite incongruous. Remember, Serena Williams is considered overweight or obese, as are many athletes, simply because they carry more muscle mass. We are born with a certain body type, which we can't change but only manage through exercise and eating properly. It is possible to be healthy and fit with any body type and shape.

While there are 3 distinct body type categories, we don't fall into just one category. Most people are a mix of two or all three body types. However, most people do have dominant traits from one. Think of an individual like Jennifer Lopez. She is predominantly an endomorph with the larger buttocks and thighs, but has some traits of the mesomorph as well, like a smaller waist.

Here are characteristics and examples of the three different *body types*:

Ectomorph

If you are an ectomorph, you have an advantage over most people when it comes to being thin. Long, lean muscles and limbs, low fat storage and a slim frame can characterize ectomorphs.

Individuals with this body type are called hard gainers. If you have this body type you will have less of a struggle with being overweight. Women like Kiera Knightly, Gwyneth Paltrow and Courtney Cox are considered ectomorphic body types. Even an ectomorph can be overweight. They have small frames that look relatively thin in clothes except when they have a larger waist. When they gain weight, it is predominantly noticeable in the hips and stomach region and less noticeable in the arms and legs. Ectomorphs that do become overweight typically do so as they age and their lives become more sedentary.

Mesomorph

Mesomorphs can usually be characterized by large bones, solid torso, low fat levels, wide shoulders with a narrow waist. Mesomorphic refers to the squareness or muscularity of the physique, resulting from an excess of muscle over the other components. Individuals with this body type are generally lean and muscular. Mesomorphs gain muscle easily but would not tend to gain fat. Women like Demi Moore and Jessica Simpson would be considered mesomorphs.

Very few women are pure mesomorphs. They tend to also have features that include either the ectomorph or the endomorph body type. Mesomorphs can also become overweight especially if unhealthy lifestyles and poor eating habits exist. The weight gain for the mesomorph would be in the upper body and waist area.

Endomorph

If you are big boned, have extra junk in the trunk, or gain ten pounds by simply looking at an éclair, then you are probably an endomorph. Endomorphs are characterized by increased fat storage, a wide waist and a large bone structure. This body type causes the most problems with weight gain. The endomorphic body type refers to the component of roundness in the physique, produced most often by an excess of fat over muscle. The structure of this body type exhibits an emphasis on the stomach and the gut. The endomorphic body type has the greatest difficulty in managing body fat. Endomorphs gain body fat the easiest and struggle the greatest to keep excess weight off. However, this is not to say that an endomorph can't be in shape and fit. In fact, if a quality nutrition and exercise plan is followed, this body type can gain muscle size and strength easier than the other two body types. Women like Jennifer Lopez, Kate Winslet and Queen Latifah would be considered endomorphic.

I can hear all the endomorphs, including myself, saying, "But I don't look like Jennifer Lopez." Well, if you had millions of dollars and access to her personal chefs and trainers, you probably would. If some of these celebrities were working middle class moms, with 3 kids, a job and were the designated chauffeurs for all sports and after school activities, they would probably weigh a few extra pounds more, too. Possibly 40 or 50 pounds more.

Interestingly, there appears to be a correlation with the endomorphic body type and weight bias. It may be because of the rounder and softer look of this body type, or the fact that more fat is generally stored in the waist or hip areas. There are a significantly less number of celebrities in the media that have an endomorphic body type. So when it comes to weight bias, it is more about the appearance of being obese rather than actually being obese. Even when you see someone overweight in Hollywood, it is typically either an ectomorph or mesomorph that has gained weight rather that an individual that is an endomorph.

The media was really rough on actress Patricia Arquette (who would be considered a mesomorph body type) about her weight gain after her pregnancy. But even with the little bit of added weight, she was by no means fat. Could you imagine how ruthless they would be to an endomorphic woman in the same situation? Weight bias against endomorphic body types is similar to the bias exhibited toward the obese in general (even if the endomorph is not technically obese). If body fat percentage would become the actual gauge of health, rather than the height-weight chart, then scales and numbers on a scale really become obsolete. What woman wouldn't cheer for that day?

Endomorph Extra

While no fad diet works, endomorphs typically do better on nutritional plans that are lower in carbohydrates. This is because endomorphs tend to be sensitive to carbohydrates. This means when you eat carbohydrates it causes a spike in insulin, which requires your body to release a lot of insulin to lower blood sugar levels. This inhibits fat burning and increases fat storage. If you eat meals with a lot of carbohydrates and feel like you're ready to go into hibernation, then you are probably sensitive to carbohydrates - typical for an endomorph.

Any body type can become overweight or obese. However, endomorph body types are genetically predisposed to carry extra weight. This doesn't mean endomorphs can't maintain a healthy weight; it just means they may have to work a little harder than the other body types. The good news is that this body type also has a tendency to carry weight in all the right places, which some women would kill for as well. While endomorphs seem to receive the brunt of bias, none of the body types are excluded. Nevertheless, it is important to remember that endomorphs have many positive attributes. Endomorphs tend to be friendly, extraverted, tolerant, calm natured and goal oriented.

Here are a few extra tips that are even more relevant for the endomorph body type. If you've tried everything and still carry a few extra pounds, take these thoughts into consideration:

- Keep your nutrition simple. If you eat the same foods daily, like many athletes, then your body actually becomes more efficient at burning the foods.
- Eat protein with every meal. Intake 25-30% of calories in protein.
- Since endomorphs are generally insulin resistant, or carbohydrate sensitive, then it is best to consume carbohydrates with only one or two meals per day.
- Snacks should be low in carbohydrates. Snacks should also include protein, such as cheese, peanut butter, nuts or even meat.
- Keep cheat meals to two or less per week. Make sure the meals contain adequate protein.
- Many endomorphs are people persons. The problem with being a social butterfly is that working out can be a very isolating activity. I hate to walk on a treadmill alone, but I love to go for a walk with friends. Endomorphs should exercise with others or participate in activities where there is also a social aspect, such as group fitness classes.
- Endomorphs tend to be goal oriented. This can be great as far as setting goals for motivation to get healthy. However, when results do not come as quickly as may be expected then it can become an excuse to give up. Therefore, set realistic goals so that you feel successful and desire to continue.
- Endomorphs are hard wired to avoid discomfort. I, for one, love when everything is comfortable and relaxing. However, this makes it difficult to push through barriers to improve fitness. This is one reason you may have given up on fitness in the past. However, remember it is baby steps. Start with an easy and quick workout and then build on it.
- Endomorphs may be insecure about working out. Compared to other body types, endomorphs may lack confidence and self-esteem. This may keep you out of the gym or fitness class. So go with a friend, or find a different activity to engage in, but the key is to get healthy and get moving any way you can.

There is No Ideal Shape

As there is no ideal weight, there also is no ideal body shape, despite what magazines and the media have claimed for ages. As soon as we figure that out, we'll feel a lot better about wearing our favorite jeans out for a night on the town. Ideal is not a body shape; ideal is healthy. And whether that makes you a size 2 or a size 14, provided you're living a well-balanced and active lifestyle, you should embrace your natural tendencies and relish in taking care of yourself.

There is also a tremendous gap between what women think is ideal and what men think is ideal. Men prefer women with more curves than a stick. Part of the reason is genetically driven, where men are attracted to women who appear fertile and able to reproduce. When men see women with a little "ba-donka-donk," they are more likely to find them appealing, not repulsive.

Not only do you have a distinct body type, as we've discussed earlier, but you also have a distinctive body *shape*. It is based on the size of your physical features and the overall balance of your body. Where you tend to naturally store body fat is also based upon your body shape. There are four main body shapes that are derived from body type: *Banana, Apple, Pear,* and *Hour Glass*. The fashion industry loves the thin shape, which is considered Banana. The Hour Glass is perceived as having the greatest sex appeal. Like the body types, we can actually be a combination of body shapes, but typically one shape is dominant. It is good to know and understand your body shape in regards to how you should train or eat.

A study by North Carolina State University examined the shapes of American women:

46% are described as rectangular or Banana shape (with a waist less than nine inches smaller than the hips or bust). 22% of women are bottom-heavy or Pear shaped (hips two inches or more larger than bust). 14 % of women are inverted triangles, busty or Apple shaped (bust is three or more inches bigger than hips). 8% of women are Hour Glass shaped (bust and hip measurements are equal).

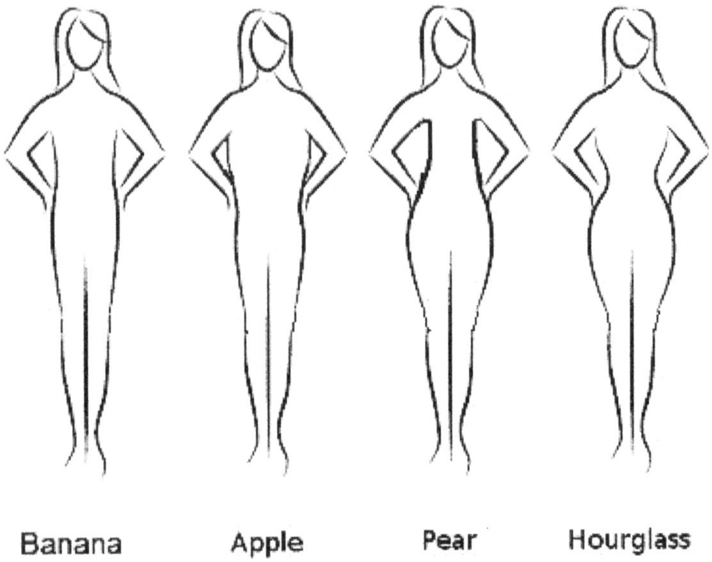

Here are characteristics associated with each body shape:

Banana: Mostly an ectomorph body type. The waist is less than nine inches smaller than the hips or bust. Body fat is distributed predominantly around the waist. They have a narrow bust and narrow hips. Some call this body type a ruler shape or even a pencil shape. Examples of this body type include Cameron Diaz and Gwyneth Paltrow.

Hour Glass: Most likely either mesomorph or endomorph body type. Tend to have equal hip and bust measurements with a narrow waist. Body fat distribution tends to be around both the upper body and lower body. Body fat distribution starts with the arms, breasts, hips and rear before any other parts including waist and upper abdomen. Considered by many as the body shape that is desired. The bust and the buttocks are nicely proportioned while the waist is thin, thus giving the body an appearance of the hourglass. Examples of this body shape would be Scarlett Johansson, Jessica Alba, Halle Berry and Kim Kardashian.

Apple: Most likely either mesomorph or endomorph body type. Bust is bigger than hips. Body fat distribution tends to begin in the arms, shoulders, chest and upper abdomen first. Apple shape tends to describe women who have wide torsos (full bust, waist and upper back), as they store body fat around the mid section of their bodies (stomach, abdomen and chest). Such women have relatively slim thighs and upper legs. Apple shaped women often have a top-heavy appearance, with a bust and midriff bigger than the hips, a prominent stomach and flat buttocks. Examples of this shape would be Dolly Parton, Tyra Banks, Demi Moore, Teri Hatcher and Catherine Zeta-Jones.

Pear: Mostly an endomorph body type. The hip measurement is larger than the bust. Pear shaped generally describes women who store fat below the waistline on the hips, thighs and buttocks (as opposed to their stomachs and midsections). As body fat percentage increases, an increasing proportion of body fat is distributed around the waist and upper abdomen. Such fat being stored on the thighs often leads to cellulite. Examples of this body shape include Jennifer Love Hewitt and Kate Winslet.

You Can Be Skinny and Still Be Fat

Despite what *Free To Be You (And Me)* attempted to teach us from the tender age of pre-teen, we quickly learned that to be tall and slim was *ideal*, leaving anyone with curves or an *average* build to try their hand at dieting or to go on an exercise craze. And while it's important to eat balanced meals and to live an active lifestyle, it should be for good health and good health alone – not to squeeze into a size two strapless dress. As soon as you begin comparing yourself to anyone, it's a dangerous game that never ends - until you decide to embrace your natural self and enjoy a well-balanced lifestyle.

"Being thin doesn't automatically mean you're not fat," said Dr. Jimmy Bell, a professor of molecular imaging at Imperial College, London. Since 1994, Bell and his team have scanned nearly 800 people with MRI machines to create *fat maps* showing where people store fat. According to the data, people who maintain their weight through diet rather than exercise are likely to have major deposits of internal fat, even if they are otherwise slim. "The whole concept of being fat needs to be redefined," said Bell, whose research is funded by Britain's Medical Research Council. He further suggests that without a clear sign, like an oversized waist, individuals may falsely assume they are healthy.

What this research explains is that skinny people can still be fat. When you starve yourself, you are actually losing muscle mass. So you can look smaller but you will still carry excess fat internally, Dr Bell suggests. Unfortunately, many celebrities have dealt with anorexia such as the singer Karen Carpenter, Tracy Gold, Candace Cameron and many others including gymnast Christy Henric, who in 1988 was told by a U.S. judge that she had to lose weight in order to make the Olympic team. As a result of anorexia, she died of multiple organ failure. She was only 22 years of age.

Individuals who are very skinny but have little muscle mass are known as skinny-fat. That means they basically have skeleton, fat and skin. You have probably seen very skinny people who didn't appear to have any muscle tone. In fact, one fashion photographer commented that when he touched a model's arm it was "spongy." This can be attributed to her body fat, even though she was skinny.

Experts have long known that fat, active people can be healthier than their skinny, inactive counterparts. "Normal-weight persons who are sedentary and unfit are at much higher risk for mortality than obese persons who are active and fit," said Dr. Steven Blair, an obesity expert at the University of South Carolina. Think about the super-sized Sumo wrestlers. They probably have a better metabolic profile than some of their slim, sedentary spectators. The reason that's possible is because the wrestlers' fat is primarily stored under the skin, not streaking throughout their vital organs and muscles.

Finally, research suggests that being slightly overweight is actually healthier than being underweight, especially if the underweight person is not physically active. People who are underweight may not receive adequate nutrition, which means they are more susceptible to sickness, have a weakened immune system and may not be able to recover from injuries. They may also have less muscle mass and be susceptible to osteoporosis.

This knowledge is overlooked by the media and even by most experts in the health field. More important than your weight or even your body fat is how your body fat is distributed in your body. Skinny people can actually have a higher body fat percentage than a larger person. If someone is anorexic or dieting to the point where they lose more muscle than body fat, then they are skinny-fat. These individuals aren't healthy or fit. Yet, they don't look fat, so they don't endure the same kind of bias as people who do look fat.

Curvy is Not Plus-Sized

Curves come in all shapes and sizes, but cultural bias and the media would have us believe that curvy really means plus-sized. Hollywood tries to convince us that there are only two ideal body shapes, stick thin and hourglass (but their emphasis is definitely on stick thin). As far as the hourglass shape, a bigger chest or derriere doesn't necessary equate to being curvy or plus sized.

Ingrained weight bias pushes our culture to create an ideal shape that is not realistic. The fashion industry now considers a size 6 to be plus-sized. This poses the question and concern about what is realistic, safe and attractive for women in today's culture. According to an ABC News report, twenty years ago there was an 8% disparity between the average woman and the average fashion model. Today that disparity is up to 23%.

The media, print magazine and fashion designers are creating an unattainable image for impressionable young girls, teens and even adult women. The negative connotation associated with the term *Plus Size* places incredible pressure on women. Now more than ever, women need positive reinforcement that they are beautiful. With so many negative forces weighing on us, we need praise, encouragement and confidence. We're working against forces every day that are negative. For example, twenty years ago the average fashion model was a size 8. Today, the average fashion model is an emaciated size 0. (Meanwhile, during those same two decades, the average

American woman, who stands 5' 4" expanded from a size 10 to a size 14.)

However there is good news, men are less influenced by the media than women. A research study concluded that when given a choice, men prefer brown-haired, blue-eyed size 14 women. That's right, a size 14! The research concluded that men in the US, UK and Australia all preferred women in the 12- 14 size range. And here we are scaring ourselves skinny for what? Certainly not to look good in the eyes of the average male, as this study suggests. Since a size 12 can be fit and fabulous, maybe that should be our goal. As opposed to a size 2, 4, 6, 8 who do we appreciate? Real women, that's who! And the real guys that love them.

The Eye of the Beholder

Yes, beauty is in the eye of the beholder. But what if our eyesight has become so skewed because of an obsession with being thin that we don't see well. If we can't really see ourselves, how can we ever accept who we are? Acceptance is the final stage of the grieving process. My question to you is how long have you been mourning your body? Have you wasted years, like I have, worrying about having the perfect figure or feeling that if you were just a certain body type, everything in your world would fall into place - you'd find that fantastic mate, get that dream job? If you had the perfect body, then what would you worry about? Growing old, crow's feet, athlete's feet? Or better yet, what if you had the perfect body and still weren't satisfied with it? What if your attitude never changed, so in your mind's eye you didn't even realize you had the perfect body?

Pressure to be thin has distorted our image of ourselves. Even if you have a nice figure, you probably think you are fat because the media only portrays women as twigs who could snap if blown by a gusty breeze. In Bravo's cable show How To Look Good Naked, they line up women according to size from smallest to largest. They then ask the contestant to decide where she thinks she would fit into the line up. The overwhelming majorities think they are much bigger than they actually are, and place themselves in the larger end of the line-up. That is a powerful example of distorted self-image, something quite normal for many of us.

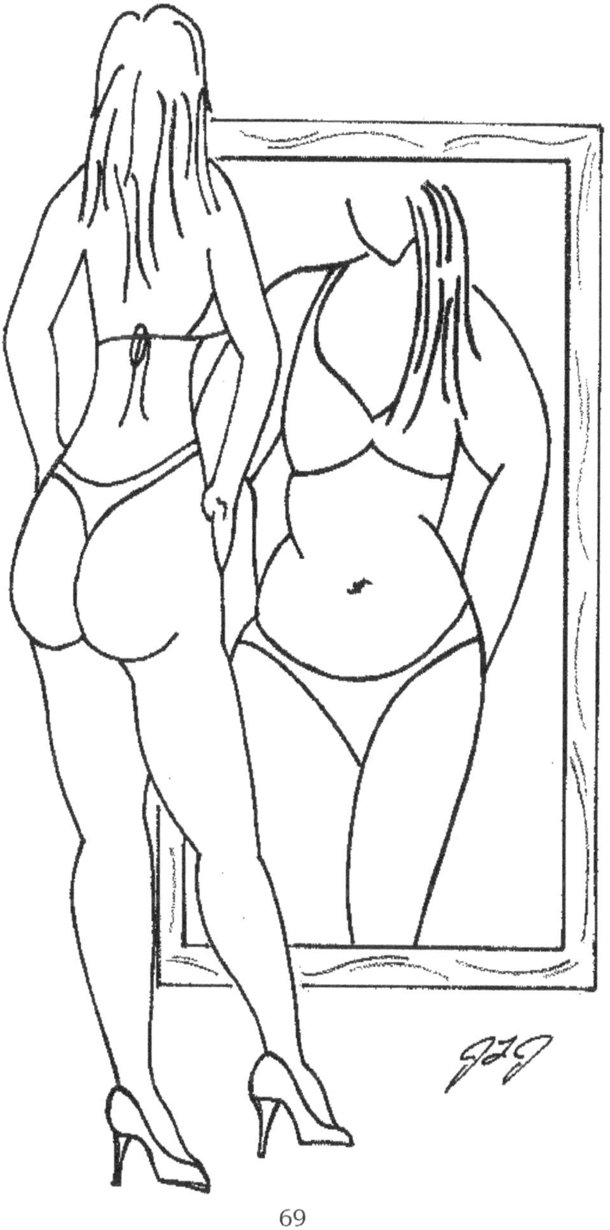

Will we ever be content with our bodies? Even if other people thought you had a perfect body, would you still see only its flaws? Will you spend the rest of your life in a frustrated attempt to live up to unrealistic expectations or will you finally learn to love yourself, embrace your health and strive to live with an acceptance that you were made the way you are for a purpose. Whether you are 4'9" or you are 6'1", you can be healthy and happy. Strive for this state of mind and see how quickly your body suddenly appears more perfect than you ever dreamed possible.

The Endomorph Diaries

I was given my first diary when I was 12 years old. My grandmother bought it for my birthday that year. It was one of my favorite gifts.

My dear grandmother always struggled with her weight. I can remember, even back then, how grandma would diet, rip out weight loss articles from magazines and hang them on the fridge. I always knew whenever grandma was dieting because there would be cottage cheese in her refrigerator. And I remember, even at 12 years old, writing about how I wished I was thin like Caroline Karavas, the popular girl in school. How I yearned to be *normal,* like her.

Recently I was cleaning out a closet and found my old diaries. I took an afternoon off, drank many cups of tea and read them all. I was stunned by what was important to me back then - things that seem so very trivial now. I noticed throughout all my diaries that there was always one recurring theme - *getting skinny.* As the years progressed, so did I thankfully. No longer were the burning schoolgirl questions raised – Will he call? Why didn't he call? Should I call him? Even better yet, no more wondering when I would reach my goal weight and how. Instead, there was a shift. The obsessive thinking, especially about my weight, began to subside. It happened after experiencing a profound moment on what was an otherwise ordinary day. It changed my life and upon re-reading, changed it once again. My wish is that it may do the same for you.

Below is an entry from my diary. The names have been changed to protect the innocent but the title remains the same. I've named it *Happiness is a Choice.* Dear reader, may I introduce you to my dear diary.

~~~~~~~~~~~~~~~~~~~~~~

I really wish I could look like Doreen. She is perfect - a tall, tanned, blond, blue-eyed beach babe with a figure to die for. A real hourglass 36-24-36 body that could look good in a potato sack. Miss Perfect I call her in my head. When I'm working out at the gym, sweat stinging my eyes, I pretend I am Miss Perfect. I see myself walking barefoot on the Jersey shore, strolling past the boardwalk; jeweled flip-flops dangling from my nicely manicured hand, wearing sparkling white shorts and matching top.

I have all sorts of fun as Doreen. I imagine myself in Greece, walking the hills of the Acropolis, not struggling at all with the rugged terrain and the 104-degree heat because I am in shape and impeccable in my sparkling white shorts and matching top. Life would be good as Miss Perfect. I wouldn't have any problems. How could someone have problems with a body like that? And even if there were a few, I'd be feeling too good to notice.

I spent this past weekend with Doreen. We were vacationing poolside, sipping one too many colorful frozen drinks when she says, "I just hate my body. If only I could be 30 pounds skinnier I'd be so happy." I almost choked on my wooden umbrella. "But you don't have 30 pounds to lose," I said.

She glared with the intense focus of a cat hunting her prey. "Are you kidding me? Look at this!" She pounds a fist into her thighs, then points to her arms, stomach, butt and just about every body part except for her eyelids. "Look at this.... this is huge, and here, this is really huge. Look, I could lose 10 pounds here alone. This is just disgusting."

I promptly tell her she needs her head examined. "If I looked like you, I'd be so happy." She retaliates, "If I was 30 pounds skinnier, *I'd* be so happy."

Then there was silence.

It was awkward.

It was pregnant.

It was... silent.
~~~~~~~~~~~~~~~~~~~~~~

That's when I had an epiphany. I questioned my very existence. If I looked like Doreen, would I want to be 30 pounds skinnier, too? Well maybe, just maybe. I realize that it has nothing to do with weight anymore, or size, or how good one looks. It has to do with what is in your mind.

Best way I can describe it is - a mindset - and the mindset is called *miserable.*

Yes, there are women with gorgeous, glowing, healthy bodies that are miserable. Complaining, always wanting to be something they are not. There she is, perfect and miserable.

Could my perfect be someone else's misery?

Could possibly my misery be someone else's perfect?

And if so, when are we ever happy?

Just then, a woman fatter than me walked past us in a bikini. Cellulite billowing out the sides as she chases her 4 year-old - belly hanging over belly, hanging over belly, hanging over bikini bottom. She lifted her daughter into the air and gave her a great big kiss. They were laughing and playing and eating. I mean this woman was just loving life; bikini and all. She was curvaceous, even downright overweight, but she didn't let that affect her. She was happy, having a grand old time. My first thought was - I'd be so embarrassed walking around like that. But then, on second glance, I noticed a confidence about her, a real beauty. She was perfect in her own way. Her inner beauty was shining through every move.

And then there was me and my friend. (Me, who works out every day just to maintain this level of chubbiness— and my flawless friend who lifts a gallon of milk and develops bicep muscles.) There we are: Miss Perfect and I - miserable- having a pity party, complaining on life.

There was much to learn in that moment. I realized that there is miserable curvaceous and happy curvaceous. I realized that some of us would never be satisfied, no matter what we weigh. I realized that some of us could be happy no matter what we weigh.

It's not the weight – it's me.

I can be a happy-me, simply by accepting the curves I own.

Or I can be a miserable-me, unaccepting of the curves I reject. The interesting thing is –whichever one I choose, I am still going to be me. As Billy Joel sings, "Either way it's okay, you wake up with yourself." So why shouldn't I choose to be happy?

Yes, the other day at the pool, with the little wooden umbrella in my drink, I've come to realize that happiness and self-love is a choice.

All I have to do is choose it.

From here on in, I choose *Happy*.

He was always Snow White's favorite, too.

~~~~~~~~~~~~~~~~~~~~

Weighing In (Not)

There is no ideal weight. There is no ideal body shape. Curves are normal and do not make you plus size. Women are embarrassed by their curves because the media portrays an average sized woman as plus sized. Men prefer real women; if this were not the case then no one would be dating or getting married. So, stop worrying about your shape, curves, butt and boobs. You were created with a certain body shape, which you have very little control over. The only aspect you do have control over, short of surgery, is to stay active and make your body shape one that is also healthy.

The scale will never change your body shape. If you are an endomorph, then you will never be stick thin. However, if you are an ectomorph, you probably will never have the curves that you may desire either. All you can do is work with what you have. With our newfound knowledge gleaned from this chapter (along with a peek into the diary of a former wanna-be Hour Glass who is really a Pear), I believe we can move toward ultimate health, balanced lifestyles and self-acceptance. All we can be is the best we can be. I can never be the best you. You seem to have that covered well.
~~~~~~~~~~~~~~~~~~~~

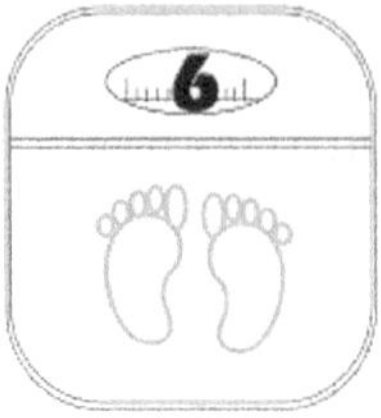

Cows are Vegetarians

When did vegetarianism become in vogue for dieting? And honestly, have you ever noticed how vegetarians focus so much on meat? They won't order meat, but they'll order stuff that reminds them of meat - veggie burgers, soy sausage, soy bacon. Meat imposters, as I like to call them. It seems they still want everything to look like meat, as if maybe they can fool their tummies into believing. Funny, I've never heard someone order a steak and ask for it to look like arugula.

Vegetarians will explain how animals such as the giraffe are vegetarians. But did you know that cows and pigs are vegetarians too? Yes, big fat cows and dirty porky pigs are vogue vegetarians! Really now, if we have to mimic an animal in nature, I would prefer we mimic a lion. Look at the female lion: she is powerful and in charge. She also is not a vegan. If we want to play the game *Which Animal Would You Be*, I'd rather be a lioness over a cow any day. How often have you heard someone called a fat lion?

Does it make sense to snub meat? It's an interesting debate. Like many herbivores, the cow has to eat slowly all day long and has more than one stomach to digest cellulose by a fermentation process. If you have a couple of extra stomachs inside of you and you have time to sit on the couch all day and digest food, then maybe you could be a vegetarian. However, the meat-eating lioness doesn't have time to sit around all day. She is busy providing food for her children and her husband - who by the way is too lazy to hunt, but thinks that he is king or something. Fortunately, the lioness can eat more infrequently and will stay well fed for a much longer period of time because of her high protein intake.

So why is vegetarianism and veganism such a topic of diet? The answer is simple, because everything is a topic of diet in our diet-crazed world. And since the rise in fad dieting, vegetarianism has risen in popularity, also.

Vegetarianism: A Healthy Choice?

There are people who become vegetarian or vegan because they believe that eating a non-meat diet is healthy and they have issues with how they think animals are treated. There are many types of vegetarians. There are those who eat no meat, dairy or eggs. There are those who eat fish, some who eat eggs and dairy, and well you get the point. There are as many flavors of vegetarianism as there are flavors at Baskin Robins - which is off limits to a vegan and probably the main reason why I could never be one.

My goal is not to argue against the beliefs of vegetarians; some may be quite noble, but simply to argue vegetarianism as a healthy diet plan. I will leave issues of animal cruelty, environment and the rest for others to debate. So, is a vegetarian diet really healthy?

Soy products are one of the major staples for vegetarians. Soy provides enough protein for a vegetarian or vegan to live. However, there are issues with consuming soy products. Soy, which is almost always genetically modified, is damaging to the thyroid, can cause infertility, causes deficiencies in zinc and iron, and scoliosis in children. Recent studies suggest that soy beverages have a higher potential to cause cavities than cow's milk. Below are some of the issues associated with soy consumption from the Weston Price Foundation Soy Symposium.

Soy phytoestrogens disrupt endocrine function and have the potential to cause infertility and to promote breast cancer in adult women. Processing of soy protein results in the formation of toxic lysinoalanine and highly carcinogenic nitrosamines. Vitamin B12 analogs in soy are not absorbed and actually increase the body's requirement for B12. And B12 is often found lacking in a vegetarian diet, so this compounds the problem. High levels of phytic acid in soy reduce assimilation of calcium, magnesium, copper, iron and zinc. Soy foods contain high levels of aluminum, which is toxic to the nervous system and the kidneys.

As you can see, soy may not be that great an alternative to dairy products and may actually be very harmful. Aside from the health risk, those who attempt a meat-free diet without soy usually fail, because they cannot get enough protein.

A lack of carnosine has been noted as one of the biggest issues with vegetarians, and this is especially true with the much more extreme vegan diets. Carnosine is a dipeptide, which is critical to preventing lethal glycation reactions in the body. A lack of carnosine alters the body's proteins and renders them non-functional. While wrinkled skin is the first outward appearance of glycation, most degenerative diseases are affected in one way or another by pathological glycation reactions. Glycation is involved in disorders as diverse as cataract, cancer and Alzheimer's disease.

The problem is that carnosine is only found in meat. Some vegetarians try to compensate with supplements, but such attempts are futile due to the rate at which carnosine is used. Synthetic 50 mg supplements of carnosine, which are commonly used by vegetarians and vegans, are virtually useless - because 7 ounces of beef provides the body about 5 times that amount and is used up in 5 hours. This means carnosine supplements provide virtually no benefit to a vegetarian.

Another deficiency found in vegetarians is vitamin B-12, which is found in meats. Many vegetarians seem healthy for several years before developing problems related to B-12 deficiencies. Lack of B-12 results in a higher risk of heart disease and stroke, problems with the central nervous system (CNS), tingling in the hands and feet, fatigue, anemia and eventually can cause permanent damage including blindness, deafness and dementia. These problems are exaggerated in the elderly.

Anemia is a potentially serious condition in which the body does not make enough oxygen-bearing red blood cells. Anemia can also be problematic for vegetarians and especially women. This is usually due to an iron deficiency. Iron is available in two forms: heme and non-heme. Heme-iron is the most easily used by your body and is found in meat, poultry and fish. Supplements can be taken to increase the amount of iron in the diet, but eating meats will ensure that you are getting quality iron.

Finally, a major issue with vegetarianism is a problem that everyone faces who eats fruit and vegetables from the supermarket. Some of these foods that you think would be healthy are actually some of the worst foods that can be consumed because of chemicals and pesticides. In fact, there is what's known as *The Dirty Dozen* (no, not the movie) but rather a list of foods that have high levels of pesticides that need to be avoided. These include apples, celery, strawberries, peaches, spinach, nectarines, grapes, bell pepper, potatoes, blueberries, lettuce and kale. Two of these, apples and potatoes, are two of the most commonly consumed products. Below is a more detailed look at why they are not an ideal choice.

Apples: If all fruits held a "most doused in pesticides contest," apples would win. Why? They are individually grafted (descended from a single tree) so that each variety maintains its distinctive flavor. As such, apples don't develop resistance to pests and are sprayed frequently. The industry maintains that these residues are not harmful. But Mark Kastel, an executive at a farm-policy research group claims, "It's just common sense to minimize exposure by avoiding the most doused produce, like apples." He continues, "Farm workers have higher rates of many cancers."

Potatoes: Root vegetables absorb herbicides, pesticides and fungicides that wind up in soil. In the case of potatoes, the nation's most popular vegetable, they're treated with fungicides during the growing season, and then sprayed with herbicides to kill off the fibrous vines before harvesting. After they're dug up, the potatoes are treated yet again to prevent them from sprouting. "Try this experiment: Buy a conventional potato in a store, and try to get it to sprout. It won't," says Moyer, who is a farm director of the Rodale Institute (also owned by Rodale Inc., the publisher of Prevention).

If you have reasons other than eating healthy, you may not be persuaded to stop the vegan or vegetarian lifestyle.

But, if it is about being healthy, then the facts show that vegetarianism does not live up to its hype. In fact, there is no substantial data to show that vegetarians live longer or are healthier than their meat-eating counterparts.

Interestingly, according to *Psychology Today*, roughly 75% of vegetarians eventually return to eating meat, with 9 years being the average length of abstinence. The most common reason former vegetarians returned to meat was declining health. As one vegetarian turned omnivore stated, “I'll take a dead cow over anemia any time.” It sounds as if many people turn to vegetarianism as some kind of fad diet, which in the long run is found to be ineffective. Besides, let's be real, how many people can really give up a bacon double cheeseburger for the rest of their lives?

Organic Foods

Ah “organic,” the Greek word that means double the price. Have you seen the cost of organically grown foods in the grocery store? They are muy cara. (That's Spanish for expensive, I really don't know Greek.) But I do know that organic prices are outrageous. Unfortunately, many fruits and vegetables grown traditionally are full of chemicals and pesticides, not a healthy choice regardless of whether or not you are a vegetarian. While organic foods may be more expensive, *The Dirty Dozen* foods, which have high levels of pesticides, should be purchased as organic or avoided altogether. Your body is well worth it and it will thank you. Fortunately, there are some foods that have very low levels of pesticides such as onions, sweet corn, mushrooms, avocados, and even asparagus, which can be purchased normally. For these particular foods, it's not worth paying the extra money to buy them organic.

Even with meats and dairy, it is important to look for foods that are free of hormones and other chemicals. Many meats and dairy products have unhealthy chemicals that may lead to weight gain. Some animals are pumped full of hormones to make them grow faster and larger. However, these hormones are probably not ideal for human consumption. So, it is best to purchase meats and dairy products that are hormone and additive free. Many grocery stores are offering a greater variety of these products, which in turn makes them more affordable and a healthier choice than hormone injected products. While some fruits and vegetables have high levels of pesticides, there are still ways to get healthy produce. The best solution would be to grow your own fruit and vegetables when possible. Believe me, you don't have to be Ma and Pa Kettle to grow some nice tomatoes. If a green thumb isn't your thing, then simply try to buy from local growers, such as local farmers markets. Farmers who grow on a smaller scale typically use fewer pesticides and the foods will be fresher. Plus, you will be helping the local economy. It's a win-win situation.

Food Guide Fiasco

One of the reasons vegetarianism has gained popularity in the dieting community is because the food guidelines of the late 1970's and 1980's were created to favor a vegetarian lifestyle. It seemed to suggest that dairy and especially meat and fats were loathsome. Why is protein seen as a mere afterthought in the food pyramid? Was there extensive research that caused this to happen?

The food guide is one of the many culprits that contribute to weight gain. Most people think nutritionists or scientists who worked for the government developed the food guide. But it was actually created by a vegetarian, who apparently wanted to demonize the meat and dairy industry. So, he made carbohydrates the focus of nutrition and negated the importance of fats and protein in the diet.

USA Food Guidelines Authors had Hidden Agendas

One of the major factors in weight gain over the past several decades can be attributed to the food guideline changes that were made in the late 1970's. Let's face it; most people assume the food guidelines must be accurate since we have been following them since 1917. Originally the guidelines were called *How to Select Foods* and were authored by Caroline Hunt, a nutritionist for the USDA. The food groups recommended were:

- Milk and meat
- Cereals

- Vegetables and fruit
- Fats and fatty foods
- Sugars and sugary foods

In 1946, it was named *National Nutrition Guide.* This guide offered 7 food groups, which supported the RDA (recommended daily allowance) requirements:

- Milk and milk products
- Meat, poultry, fish, eggs, beans, peas and nuts
- Bread, flour and cereals
- Leafy green and yellow vegetables
- Potatoes and sweet potatoes
- Citrus, tomato, cabbage, salad greens
- Butter, fortified margarine

During the 1970's, the food guidelines were changed again. It began under the leadership of a senate committee led by George McGovern. However, this time it was not developed by scientists or nutritionists. Interestingly, a vegetarian named Nick Mottern, who had no scientific background or experience writing about science or nutrition, wrote these guidelines. They were called *Dietary Goals for Americans* and the recommendations were to increase carbohydrate intake to 60%, reduce fat intake to 30% or less (with 10% or less coming from saturated fat) and reduce protein intake to approximately 10% of total calories. What a stark contrast from the previous guidelines that included fats and meats.

What caused this shift in the guidelines? Was there extensive research that prompted the change? No. Apparently Mottern, along with McGovern and others on the senate committee, decided that meat and fats were dangerous and therefore recommended limiting fat intake, which meant limiting meat and dairy products as well. At the time, very few people were in favor of the recommendations and many experts believed that the guidelines were simply being pushed on the public. In fact, many in the scientific community viewed this agenda as a nefarious attempt to destroy the meat and dairy industries.

Does this sound like credible scientific research? Hardly. And why was McGovern's committee even in charge of the guidelines? McGovern had originally formed the committee to eradicate hunger and malnutrition in the US. But as the funding began to run out, he basically decided to make changes to the food guidelines so that funding would continue for his committee! Ah, politics at its best. As Gary Taubes writes in his article *The Soft Science of Dietary Fat*: "It was Senator George McGovern's bipartisan, non legislative Select Committee on Nutrition and Human Needs--and, to be precise, a handful of McGovern's staff members, that almost single-handedly changed nutritional policy in this country and initiated the process of turning the dietary fat hypothesis into dogma."

The guidelines weren't steeped in scientific validity, but rather many agencies and scientists actually refuted the claims put forth by Mottern in the McGovern report. However, it was finalized by the efforts of the committee to push it through quickly and quietly, and thus it became the country's new guidelines. The changes that were put in place drastically transformed the percentages of intake for fats, carbohydrates and protein. With a stroke of the pen, they have altered how Americans have eaten for the past 30 years. This one event went on to become a major contributor in today's weight epidemic. This is so egregious and I find it maddening. It must never be forgotten that one of the major reasons for weight gain over the past 3 decades was due to manipulation by a government agency and manipulation by individuals with a hidden self-serving agenda, which went on to have pervasive negative effects on our culture.

Weighing In

The problems with the guidelines are twofold. First, they were developed with the intent of demonizing or at least minimizing the meat and dairy industry. Secondly, the guidelines were never designed as requirements needed for active people. For most of us, the percentages of nutrients in our diet should be approximately 40-50% carbohydrates, 25-30% protein and 25-30% fats. These are the percentages that will allow for optimal nutrition.

It seems that our great grandparents may have been smarter than we have ever given them credit. They understood the importance of eating fats, carbs and protein. The problem with our contemporary food guidelines is that it focuses on removing an important nutrient from our diet. Protein. Even animals in the wild do not purposely deprive themselves of nutrients and yet we, the intelligent species, constantly deprive our bodies of what it needs to survive. A tiger doesn't shun a piece of meat and opt for a chopped salad due to cholesterol concerns.

If you do decide to choose a vegetarian lifestyle, make sure you understand how to supplement the nutrients needed so that you can achieve health and balance. And whether a vegetarian or not, be aware of your food choices and make sure you are putting needed nutrients in your body. Stay away from pesticide or hormone-laden food just like you would processed food. Simply put, your health depends upon consuming healthy foods.

In an attempt to fit an unrealistic expectation of society, we go to extremes to get thin, including consuming little more than grass hoping it will make us skinny. Yet, fad dieting and starving ourselves of vital nutrients such as protein, is abusing the very bodies that we worry so much about. We know that 75% of vegetarians eventually return to an omnivore diet. Let's face it, we didn't climb to the top of the food chain to eat algae and grass all day long.

Normally meat, dairy and eggs should be included in every meal. If a balanced diet should consist of 25-30% of protein, then this means most women aren't getting enough of it. So, one of the best things you can do beginning right now is to go and get yourself good protein. Someone once asked me the age-old question, "What came first, the chicken or the egg?" My answer, "I'll take both."

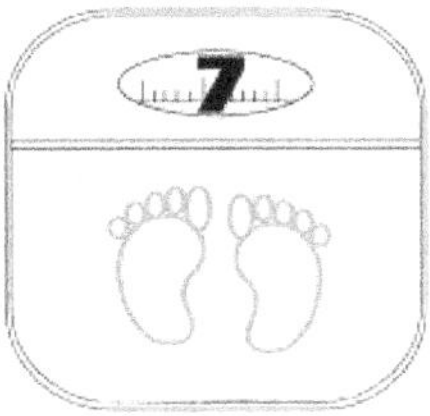

Eat Like a Champ

A recent study revealed that women on diets worry more about what they eat than their relationships. So, if given the choice between a date night with my husband or eating a calorie-free cheeseburger, I just might take the burger. Our culture creates such a fear of being overweight that we've lost our sense of priorities - and sometimes even our minds. In order to keep our sanity, we should live by this mantra: Eat to be fit. Don't starve to be skinny.

Did you ever think that eating would be one area where you could actually be like a champion? You may never run, swim or lift like a champion, but you can eat like one. This alone should be motivation enough to rethink the whole dieting phenomenon. The fittest people on earth not only eat, but eat often.

Our bodies were designed to eat like a champ; they were designed to metabolize carbohydrates, fats and proteins. Human livers were not designed to metabolize preservatives, artificial flavors, sweeteners and processed edibles. It is quite a feat of mankind that we are still functioning at this point, really.

Clean and Simple

Body builders and Olympic athletes have some of the best physiques in the world and guess what? They eat. They are not starving themselves. They know how many calories they are consuming and they eat real food. However, they don't overeat (which is important for anyone looking to improve their overall health). What do fitness and competitive athletes do different? They eat only healthy foods, which is called eating clean. And they keep their menus simple.

Sure, we have often heard you need variety in every meal. But if you look at the best physiques in the world, they tend to eat the same foods every day. This is because the body actually becomes more efficient at burning foods if they are eaten regularly. Athletes make sure their meals include fats, carbohydrates and protein. Staples of their diets are such foods as chicken, turkey, rice, potatoes and vegetables. They never do fad diets or consume diet food products. I asked a good friend who is a body builder what she thought about diet foods and she bluntly exclaimed, "They are nothing but crap, you need to eat real food!" This doesn't mean that they never have a cheat meal or enjoy a dessert, but they keep these to a minimum.

This chapter will examine the nutrients needed for a balanced diet and will offer several suggestions for various foods, such as a variety of vegetables for carbohydrates. However, this doesn't mean that you need a variety of vegetables for daily meals, but rather that you should choose a couple that you like or find works well for your body and keep them as staples in your diet. If you hate brown rice, then don't try to force brown rice into your diet. Find healthy foods you like or you won't eat them consistently. Remember the purpose of eating is to fuel your body for optimum health. If you keep it simple, consistent, and eat with purpose, you will see your body transforming into a healthy one.

Eat What You Need

While eating healthy is important, you will also need to keep track of the amount of calories you consume. If you know you need 1,500 calories per day, for example, then it will be easier to figure what foods to eat with each meal to optimize your energy needs.

Here is a formula to estimate your **basic calorie needs:**
Female: 655 + (4.3 X your weight in pounds) + (4.7 X your height in inches) – (4.7 X your age in years). This will be your basal metabolic rate.
Example: A 30 year old woman who weighs 140lbs, and is 64 inches tall.
655 + (4.3 x 140lbs) + (4.7 x 64 inches) - (4.7 x 30) = 1416 calories
So, this individual would need to consume at least 1,400 calories per day for her body to perform basic functions.

Another quick reference would be based upon body type. Simply multiply your body weight by the calories based upon your body type. This will estimate you basic caloric needs.
Ectomorph: 14 calories. Example 140 lb x 14= 1960 calories
Mesomorph: 12 calories. Example 140 lb x 12= 1680 calories
Endomorph: 10 calories. Example 140 lb x 10= 1400 calories

Most caloric formulas add calories based upon activity levels. But, if you are carrying excess weight, then stored body fat will fuel the difference. So, you should be fine with consuming the basic caloric figure, but do not drop below this amount since this is the minimum calories needed for your body's essential functions. Dropping below your basic caloric needs would be considered fad dieting and needs to be avoided.

The Body is a Machine

There are four macronutrients that your body requires in order to function properly. They are: carbohydrates, fat, protein and water. Yes, your body really does need carbs and fat. I know it sounds almost irreverent, but it's true. Your body is like a car. To run properly, a car needs fuel, oil and radiator fluid. Where our bodies are concerned, carbohydrates are fuel, fat is oil and protein is radiator fluid. Like a car, your body will not function properly without all the essential nutrients. Sure, you may drive your car for a while without oil, but it won't be for very long. And the damage caused by driving it without oil is severe - a seized engine, a damaged transmission.

If you treat your body in the same manner as our fictitious car, you could end up with no energy, consumed muscle tissue or even worse, a damaged heart. Don't treat your '08 Chevy better than you would yourself. Have you fueled up your high performance body for the work it needs to do today?

Eating clean doesn't mean you need to eat broccoli for every meal. It also doesn't mean you can never enjoy a cheeseburger (with or without good company every once in a while). However, the old adage *garbage in, garbage out* rings true when it comes to eating clean. If you want a body that provides peak performance, then you need to fuel the body to perform its best.

Brains Need Carbs

Carbohydrates have been given a bad reputation in the fad-dieting world in recent years. There are so many different Low-Carb diets that one figures there must be something to them. The problem here is that the myth has a hint of truth to it. As explained in the previous chapter, the food guidelines were set in the 1970's with an extreme view, making dairy and meats out to be dangerous. The amount of carbohydrates was inflated to create a guideline that limited dairy and meats. So, there needs to be a lower percentage of carbohydrates ingested, but this doesn't mean that a no-carbohydrate diet should be followed.

Have you ever felt fatigued, like you just wanted to lie down and had no more energy to give? This may occur after a long day, a hard workout or if you haven't eaten in several hours. This is because your body is running low on carbs. They need to be consumed with each meal and are especially critical during breakfast and post exercise meals.

Carbohydrates are also the primary energy source for the brain. Notice that you feel light headed or groggy when you haven't eaten for a long period of time? It is because your brain is not getting what it needs. It's hard enough to get our brains to function properly when they are receiving adequate nutrients, so think of the issues you can run into if you aren't giving it the carbohydrates it needs to function. Imagine yourself at the most crucial point of an important meeting, the boss asks you something, you know the answer, but you can't retrieve it through the fog.

I hate that feeling. It's like you're one apple and a slice of Muenster cheese away from a promotion.

Nutrition isn't just important in athletics, but it is also important for the academic and practical side as well. Restricting carbohydrates can deplete energy levels, compromise the quality of your day and slow brain functioning. Carbohydrates are found in whole grains, milk, vegetables, fruits and beans. Here are the various types of carbohydrates recommended for the training table:

Whole Grains are high in fiber, have moderate protein levels, are low in fat and are also a good source of complex carbs. Specific examples include millet, oats, wheat germ, barley, wild rice, brown rice, buckwheat, oat bran, cornmeal and amaranth. Any product that is made from these grains is also complex as well. Whole grain bread, bagels and pasta are examples of these.

Fruits are high in water content, fiber, vitamins and they have virtually no fat at all. Fruits packed with carbohydrates include apricots, apples, oranges, plums, pears, grapefruits and prunes.

Vegetables are high in water, low in fat, have multiple vitamins and minerals and most varieties are complex carbohydrates. Broccoli, cauliflower, eggplant, potatoes, yams, corn, carrots, onions, lettuce, celery, cucumbers, cabbage, artichokes and asparagus are all examples of these.

Legumes are a class of vegetables that include beans, peas and lentils. Legumes are a good source of complex carbohydrates. Specific examples include kidney beans, black beans, garbanzo beans, soybeans and pinto beans.

Here are some typical carbohydrates that will add much needed fuel for working brains and muscles:

Grains/Legumes	Fruits/Vegetables
Oatmeal Pasta Dry cereals (Cheerios, Kashi, Corn or Rice based cereals (Non sugary) Rice Whole wheat bread Green beans Black beans Chick peas Snow peas	Blackberries Cantaloupe Blueberries Potato Broccoli Cabbage Cauliflower *Kale – recommended Mushrooms Onion Tomato

Each gram of carbohydrates provides 4 calories of energy. Carbohydrates are primarily stored for energy in skeletal muscle. Whether you are walking, lifting weights, or jumping to a conclusion, carbohydrates are used as the primary energy source. Excess carbohydrates are stored as fat, so make sure to consume not much more than 40-50% of calories from carbohydrates. Also remember that carbohydrates from processed foods should be avoided, especially since they often are high in sugar or HFCS and high in empty calories.

For example, a baked potato that weighs 140 grams has about 140 calories, versus a serving of potato chips, which weighs only 28 grams but has 155 calories. (And that's assuming you can eat just one serving.) Not very filling, huh? It sure has a lot of calories nonetheless. When ordering meals, sometimes you'll even get chips on your plate. Since when did potato chips become a part of a well-balanced meal? Choose your carbohydrates wisely; ask for nutritious ones such as fresh or frozen vegetables over their processed counterparts. Little changes in each meal every day will boost your energy to fuel your mind and active body. How well you nourish your brain will determine how well your brain will nurture you.

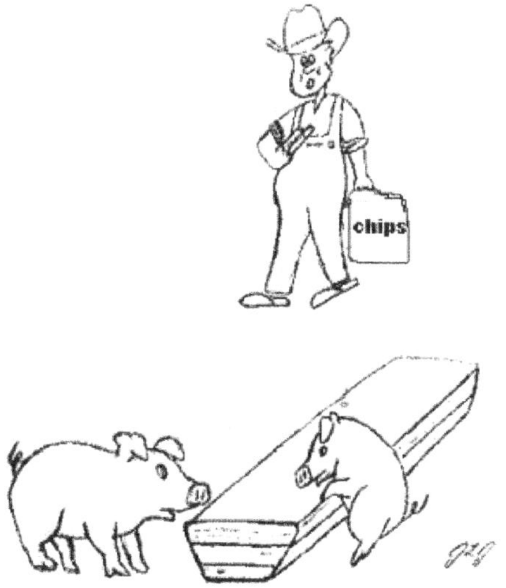

"Chips? Doesn't he know we're trying to watch our trans fats?"

Fat Gets a Bad Rap

Did you know that fat is nothing more than energy? The fat that you see on your hips and thighs when you look in a mirror is nothing more than stored energy. That idea amazes me. It's a nice way of thinking about fat. Really, my butt is just a bunch of energy I have yet to unleash? Watch out world because my butt is the bomb! Literally.

Fats are vital to a healthy and functioning body. Fat has often been given a bad rap in our diet crazy culture. With low fat diets and low fat foods prevalent in grocery stores, you would think fats should be avoided. However, stored fat provides cushion and insulation to internal organs, moves vitamins (A, D, E, and K) throughout the body and is the largest reserve of stored energy available for activity. Fat is also needed to produce hormones in the body such as testosterone and estrogen.

Fat provides the highest concentration of energy of all the nutrients. One gram of fat equals nine calories. One pound of stored fat provides approximately 3,500 calories of energy. While these calories are less accessible to performing quick, explosive activities like sprinting or weight lifting, fat is essential for longer, slower, lower intensity and endurance exercise such as easy cycling and walking. Fat also provides the main fuel source for long duration, low to moderate intensity exercise endurance sports such as cross country running or a soccer match. Even during high intensity exercise, where carbohydrates are the main fuel source, fat is needed to help access the stored carbohydrates.

There are two types of fats, saturated and unsaturated. As we know, it is not necessary to omit either from the diet. Just try not to go over the ideal 25-30% total for fats in your diet. Unsaturated fats include monounsaturated and polyunsaturated fats. These fats are typically found in plant food sources, such as olive oil. Saturated fats are found primarily in animal sources like meat, egg yolks, yogurt, cheese, butter and milk.

Since fat is slow to digest and converts into a usable form of energy (it can take up to 6 hours), it's not a good idea to eat fat immediately before or during exercise.

Here are some fats that may be part of your diet:

Avocado Canola oil Nuts Olive oil Peanut butter Macadamia nut oil-recommended	Beef Pork Eggs Cheese Sour cream

The demonization of fats, especially saturated fat, still occurs today with very little evidence in support of it. While it is best to eat more of the polyunsaturated fats such as olive oil, saturated fats do not need to be excluded from the diet altogether.

In fact, research shows that the plaque buildup in clogged arteries is approximately three-fourths unsaturated fat! Yup, believe it or not – Ripley, that is a fact. This means saturated fat is not the villainous nutrient that some would have us believe. And what about evil cholesterol? Your liver actually produces more cholesterol than you can typically eat in a day. It also tends to increase cholesterol production when you reduce its intake. Therefore, dietary cholesterol has little impact on blood cholesterol. Research suggests that if you eat healthy and are active, then fats have very little impact on your overall health.

Protein is Imperative

Protein is needed by the body to perform optimally. They are often called the building blocks of the body. Protein is made up of amino acids that combine to make muscles, bone, tendons, skin, hair and other tissues. They serve other functions as well including nutrient transportation and enzyme production.

Protein is the one nutrient that females tend to consume the least. If most women would just increase their intake of protein they would see an improved body fat ratio. Everyone should consume protein with every meal. The established guideline for protein in a sedentary person is approximately .8 grams per 2 pounds of body weight, which means about 40 grams per 100 pounds of body weight. But remember, someone who was a vegetarian established that guideline. Active individuals require more protein than a sedentary individual. Additional protein is needed for the repair of exercise-induced damage to muscle fibers, for promoting muscle growth and for facilitating the replenishment of depleted energy stores. That is why 25-30% of total calories should be consumed from proteins.

Individual requirements may vary based upon the type, size and activity level of the person. A 100-pound cross-country runner will have different protein needs than a 150-pound female who lifts weight regularly. Keep in mind that protein is not just a type of energy source, but it is needed for growth and recovery from training.

So what foods are best for consuming quality proteins? Meat and dairy products are high in protein. Beans, nuts and seeds are also good sources of protein. If you are a vegetarian, then it's important to get adequate protein from these non-meat sources or from protein shakes.

Besides beef, chicken, pork and fish, here are some examples of food high in protein:

Eggs and Dairy	Beans and Nuts
Egg, Milk, Cottage cheese, Yogurt, Soft cheeses (Mozzarella, Brie,) Medium cheeses (Cheddar, Swiss) Protein supplements (protein shakes)	Almonds Peanuts Cashews Pecans Sunflower seeds Most beans (black, pinto, lentils, etc) Soy beans

Unfortunately, there has been so much emphasis placed upon carbohydrates and fats in dieting that the importance of protein has been all but buried. Organs and the immune system are made up of protein. Even some hormones like insulin are protein based; therefore it is vital for all growth and development. Last but definitely not least, protein uses a lot of energy to digest, so consuming it actually speeds up your metabolism! Isn't that wonderful? This means your body burns more calories when you eat protein. What splendidly good news. You can be sure I'm going to have some with every single meal, including snacks. Protein. My magic ingredient for weight loss.

Water: The Forgotten Nutrient

We can potentially live for several weeks without food, but only a couple of days without water. Water is the most important nutrient of all. Since water doesn't supply actual energy, its importance in nutrition is often overlooked. It's like the stepchild of nutrients.

Water is needed for most functions in the body, including delivering oxygen, digesting food and chemical reactions. It helps get rid of waste and regulates temperature. If you experience dehydration of only 1 -2% of body weight, it can reduce strength and endurance and cause the body to work less efficiently.

While water is essential to the body, this doesn't mean you have to carry around a plastic jug of water wherever you go, or drink so much you need to find a restroom every 20 minutes. You should drink enough to remain fully hydrated. Excessive water consumption, known as water intoxication, occurs when excess water dilutes the sodium level in the bloodstream and causes an imbalance of water in the brain. This can lead to swelling of the brain and even cause death. So, too much water can potentially be dangerous.

Active individuals may need to replenish more water during exercising or sports activity. If the training takes longer than 2 hours, then they may also need to add some carbohydrates by drinking sports drinks such as Gatorade. During and after training in high temperatures, it is important to drink enough water to replenish the same amount of water that was lost. Re-hydration will help avoid cramping, heat related symptoms and decrease pain. It is critical to rehydrate the body so that it is functioning at an optimal level. Here is a guideline on hydrating amounts for an intense exercise session or an event such as a 5k run.

Preparing for Training/Activity:

2 hours before event	After event
2 cups water	2 cups water
	1/2 cup cool (45-55 degrees) water
During event	2 cups fluid for each pound lost
Every 10-15 minutes 1 cup water	Drink fluids frequently (it may take 36 hours to rehydrate completely).

While water is the most important nutrient, there is no scientific evidence that suggests everyone should drink 8-12 glasses of water each day. Besides, a glass isn't a standard measure of unit, so drinking from an eight ounce glass would provide much different results than drinking from a twenty ounce glass. A good starting point would be about 40 ounces per day. If you are active, then increase it to about 6 (8 oz) cups of water per day and if you still feel thirsty add more water throughout the day. The key here is to drink enough water, but not so much that you actually flush certain minerals and vitamins out of the body. In fact, you should start your day with 2 glasses of cold water. It will stimulate your metabolism, wake up your internal organs and get you going as well. Bottoms up!

Getting Salty Over Sodium

The scientific community has demonized sodium, like fat. Sodium actually occurs in small amounts in natural foods. However, salt is added in large quantities to processed food products. One of the main sodium ingredients is sodium benzoate, which is a type of salt created in a laboratory near you. Sodium such as sodium benzoate is used to preserve foods for a longer shelf life and it gives the food more flavor. So yes, eating processed foods is not a good idea for balancing sodium intake.

One point that is often forgotten is the relationship between sodium and potassium. Both are responsible for regulating fluid levels within the body, as well as controlling nerve impulses. Potassium actually plays an important role in regulating blood pressure with sodium. However, processed foods are typically low in potassium, yet natural foods tend to have higher potassium content. This is yet another reason to eat natural foods.

Let's look at the chart below for sodium contents in different foods:

Natural foods	**Sodium (mg)**	**Processed foods**	**Sodium (mg)**
Potato, baked	8	Burger King, large French fries (5.6oz)	940
Hamburger Broiled	60	Big Mac	1,010
Grilled Chicken	65	Grilled Chicken Club Sandwich	1,690
Beans no salt 1cup	2	Canned beans 1 cup	873
Mushrooms raw	3	Mushrooms canned	660
Onion, raw	5	Onion rings	225

Do you see what I see? Wow. Processed foods are brimming with much more sodium than our bodies were designed to utilize. If these foods were to be consumed in one day, the difference in sodium intake would be 145 mg for natural foods vs. 4500 mg for processed foods. This is just one of a quadrillion reasons why processed foods need to be consumed sparingly or avoided altogether.

The myth buster regarding sodium - it is not sodium alone that causes issues. It's the imbalance created in the body by not eating natural foods. Potassium occurs in much higher levels within natural foods such as vegetables and fruit. The exact opposite is true for sodium. Therefore, if you are consuming mainly processed foods, you may be getting too much sodium and not enough potassium in your diet. It is this imbalance between sodium and potassium that may be a factor in hypertension, not just sodium alone. Some foods you should incorporate in your diet that are high in potassium are bananas, lima beans, milk, raisins, yogurt, tomatoes and Popeye's favorite - (sorry, not fried chicken) spinach.

All Calories are Not Equal

When we look at HFCS, trans fats, saturated fats, simple sugars, proteins and different body types, it is clear that not all calories are created equal. Do you really think that the 200-calorie Twix bar sitting in the rack at the check out counter for a year affects your body the same way a 200-calorie chicken breast would? Not in the slightest, my friend. If we were having this debate in the year 1922, during a flapper convention (which I highly doubt since Twix Bars didn't even exist back then), you might be able to assert that a calorie is a calorie. But to say that now, with the invention of processed food products, is not only naïve, but is actually part of the problem we have in dealing with the weight epidemic in our culture. Which calories are bad? As we've learned in a previous chapter, most prepackaged foods are what we call food products. If it is an item that wasn't available 100 years ago, then it probably shouldn't be available today.

There are also differences in the calories of fats, carbohydrates and protein. The body must use energy to digest, absorb and metabolize the food we consume. The body uses different amounts of energy to process fats, carbohydrates and protein. Generally, more energy is required to process protein than carbohydrates, and more energy is required to process carbohydrates than fat. What this means effectively is that a 2,500-calories-a-day high-protein diet adds fewer calories to the body than a 2,500-calories-a-day high-carb diet, which in turn adds fewer calories to the body than a 2,500-calories-a-day high-fat diet. This is why increased protein is important in a well balanced diet. The key to a good body is to eat the correct ratio of nutrients and the necessary calories.

Snack Attack

Besides the food guidelines, one of the biggest influences on weight gain over the past two decades is snacking. In theory, it sounds like a good idea to eat a small amount of food between meals because it will deter overeating with meals. And actually the snacking itself may not be that bad, but it is the types of foods that are eaten that cause the problem with snacking. Most snacks are either processed foods, or predominantly carbohydrates, which might promote weight gain, rather than weight balance. If you aren't prone to snack, then don't snack just because you think it is necessary. Certain body types, such as endomorphs, have slower metabolisms, which means they shouldn't really need snacks. However, if you do get hungry occasionally between meals, then keep the following tips in mind. Do not eat snacks that are processed, like chips, cookies or even soda. Secondly, never eat snacks that have only carbohydrates. It is ideal that a snack be high in protein.

Snacking hinders weight loss if done incorrectly. Let's look at some healthy choices when packing a snack so that we can eat more often and not gain weight.

Bad snack choices	**Good snack choices**
Potato chips Cookies Fast Food Burger Ice cream Candy bar French fries Sodas Donuts	Popcorn Yogurt w/ fruit Nuts Broiled burger on whole wheat Serving of string cheese Milk Any high protein source

Eat if you are hungry; otherwise wait until your next meal. When you do snack, make sure it is predominantly protein or at least mixed with a protein, such as an apple with cheese. If you are eating 4 or 5 smaller meals per day, then these aren't the same as snacks, and each small meal should include the right mix of fats, carbs and protein.

Weighing In

By thinking of food differently, subtly but profoundly we are shifting to a new paradigm. Use this book as food for thought. When we think of food as fuel we become more inclined to ensure that the fuel we ingest is of optimal value. Food is often seen as the enemy in the battle of the bulge. In reality, food actually helps in weight management. Eating healthy meals every few hours is important to maintaining a fit body. Consuming protein with every meal and snack is important to weight management, especially for women.

However, understand that it is okay to splurge and eat a Big Mac or a Taco Grande every once in a while, so enjoy it. Eat it consciously and don't feel guilty. I once had the pleasure of watching a Zen Buddhist Monk eat his meal. It took him 15 minutes to eat a banana, a piece of cantaloupe and two grapes. He looked at it, prayed over it, gave thanks for it, stared at its pretty colors, put it to his nose and smelled each bite. He chewed each morsel in complete awe of its texture, felt it enter his stomach and gave thanks once again for all the nutrition it was providing his body. That's beautiful. That's mindful eating. If we can do just one eighth of that, we'd be so much the better for it.

More food for thought to chew on; the children are our future. Teach them to be mindful eaters, to help with the kitchen preparation and to make healthy choices. Kids do what you do, not what you say. Be a role model for them with your actions and they will have a chance at living a life free of obesity. The key to a good life is balance. If any of us thought all we had to look forward to were carrot sticks and rice cakes, we'd be a miserable species. Enjoy the good life and enjoy your food. Bon Appetit.

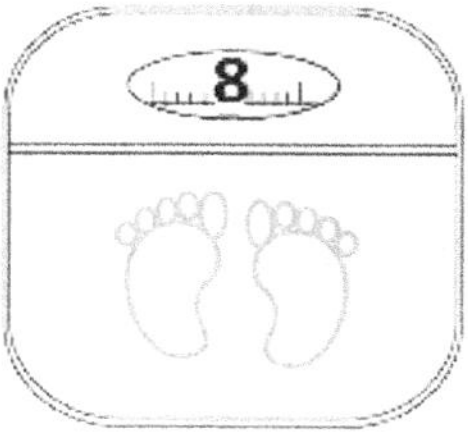

Train Like a Mother

If your focus is on being skinny, then you may end up skinny—Skinny-Fat, that is.

No, it's not a hip-hop rap artist or the latest boy band. In case you don't remember, skinny-fat refers to skinny people who are fat. It's the result of yo-yo dieting. If your focus is on dieting and not physical training, then you may never be healthy. People who diet excessively lose muscle, which causes the body to actually preserve fat as a fuel source. So while these people may lose weight, they are not losing fat. You may think Skinny-Fat sounds better than Fat (or Phat, in some cases). It's not. In fact, being skinny-fat is even unhealthier than simply being overweight.

Society is so focused on losing weight - stop thinking of it as weight loss, already. Weight loss is really a misnomer because it is not about "losing" weight so much as about burning stored energy. Weight loss would be more like walking down the street and having half of your butt fall off, now that's weight loss! But instead, the fat stored in our body is stored energy. One pound of fat has about 3,500 calories. That means you have to burn 3,500 more calories than you consume to lose one pound of body fat. So training and exercising to maintain weight is really about burning that stored energy.

Think of your metabolism as a burning fire. If you don't exercise or burn many calories during the day, then your metabolism doesn't create much of a fire. However, if you increase your metabolism (by increasing activity) then your stored body fat is actually like adding fuel to the fire. Your body will burn stored fat at a higher rate and for a

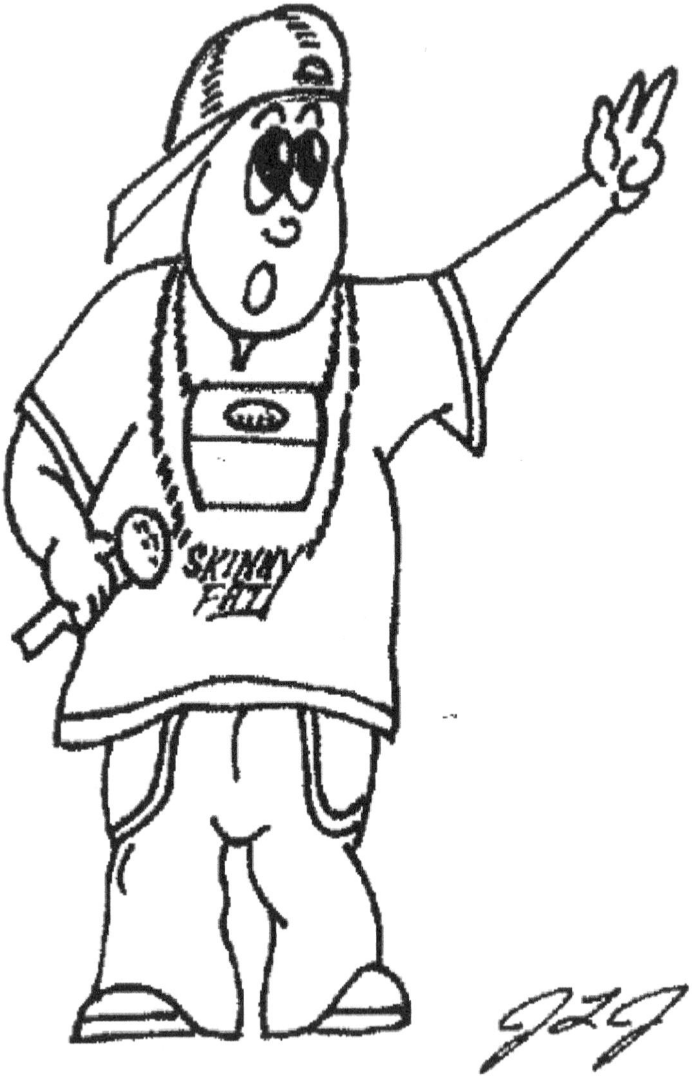

"Yo Yo Dieters in the house!"

longer period of time. So, when you combine the increased activity with the healthy eating described in the previous chapter, your body burns the stored energy (fat) much more efficiently.

Besides burning fat, increased exercise and physical activity increases growth hormone secretion, which is good for both maintaining muscle and burning fat. Increased activity also boosts metabolism for several hours after exercise, and it increases endorphins, which are also released when you binge on junk food. I'd much rather get an endorphin rush from Frisbee than from Funyuns, wouldn't you? There is much less regret.

So what does "train like a mother" mean? It means doing what mothers do best. They juggle work, home, the kids and workouts. Mothers focus most of their energy on taking care of others. I'm asking you to use that work ethic to take care of yourself, as well. You won't be able to take care of others if you don't first take care of yourself. So yes, take time to work out. "Train like a mother" is also a term indicative of women who work out quickly but with high intensity when they come to the gym. They are typically moms who know they only have a short amount of time to train before they are beckoned back to duty. They know they don't have much time to spend in the gym, so they workout with great focus and then head back to their lives. So, even if you only have a short amount of time to work out, make sure you make the most of it. You don't have to be a mother to train like one. You just need heart and a plan. In this chapter, we will examine a variety of ways to fit exercise into your busy schedule. And because you'll be training like a mother, you will do something every day, with as much intensity and passion as you can muster. Got it, mother?

How you proceed from here will depend on your current fitness level, time availability, and willingness to make changes. When I was 120 plus pounds overweight, I can tell you that I couldn't train with high intensity. Not even medium intensity. In fact, leave out the word intensity all together. Whenever I'd try to go hard, my spirit would say yes, but my body would say, you're killing me here. Since it is always best to start slow and steady, let us focus on activities that you can fit into a busy schedule and give you a foundation on which to build your stamina and your training.

We Are More Inactive Than Anyone, Anytime, Ever

Everyone is less active than any other time in history. Now that doesn't mean there aren't overweight people who are lazy. Myths and stereotypes typically have some speck of truth to them or they wouldn't become myths. There are individuals who are lazy. You may know someone like this or you may even be this person. It is time to rethink your couch potato-hood. The body was made to move, that is why it has moving parts.

However, all of our lives have become more sedentary in the information age. Whether an individual is small, medium or large, everyone is less active than in any other time of history. (Well, except maybe the ice age, I heard things were a bit stagnant back then.) And if you think skinny people are more active, well you are wrong again. Research suggests that overweight individuals sleep less and are more active than their skinnier counterparts. However, overweight people often feel embarrassed or intimated to do activities in public.

Before I lost my weight, I in no way wanted to step foot in (or even walk past by foot, for that matter) a gym. I was extremely self-conscious and felt that my body wasn't in good enough shape to join a gym. What a catch 22 - not being in good enough shape to get into good enough shape. That's like thinking you should lose weight before you get liposuction because you don't want the doctor to see your fat thighs. (By the way, lipo is not a healthy option for weight loss.) I had to start by examining activities that I could at least tolerate.

For me it was walking around my block. A block led to a neighborhood. Ten minutes led to thirty minutes, which led to purchasing a treadmill. The treadmill then led to joining a gym. Now I bike, I spin, I weight-train and I do yoga. These are things I'd never dreamed I would do when I started with that one step around the block from my house. It was consistent, incremental baby steps that helped me to succeed.

You don't have to see the entire staircase - just take the first step. There is great power in small, consistent actions. Even a drop of water consistently flowing everyday can have the power to carve out something as wonderful as the

Grand Canyon. That one drop joins other drops - together they run over rock, smoothing them in the summer, splitting them in the winter, crafting and carving them year after year. This is how canyons are made...and lives, too.

Let's Begin, Shall We

You may not be ready to make the leap to the weight room or yoga class. But, if you are going to be active, fit and healthy, you do have to make a conscience effort to get there. A good to start is to make normal chores much more active and use them as an opportunity to burn more calories. Small changes over the course of each day increase caloric expenditure.

Here are some eye-opening examples:

Activity	**Calories expended**
Letting dog out of the back door	2
Walking the dog for 30 minutes	125
Using the auto car wash	18
Washing and waxing car for 1 hour	300
Using elevator for 3 floors	Less than 1
Walking up 3 flights	15
Shopping on-line for 1 hour	30
Shopping in mall while walking for 1 hour	200
Mowing lawn (riding) for 1 hour	176
Mowing lawn (push) for 1 hour	387

The calories expended in these simple tasks are about 227 calories for the easy tasks and the more active version of the tasks are over 1,027 calories burned. A difference of over 800 calories burned doing everyday activities. It is interesting to see how simple activities can make a difference. Did you know that if you weigh 150 pounds and watch one hour of television you burn 68 calories but if you read a book for one hour you burn 89 calories? After reading, if you were to play hide and seek with your child for an hour, you would burn another 270 calories.

Let's take the approximate 1,200 calories above, which includes the hour of play, and you have burned one third of a pound worth of calories. What would you have to do in a gym to burn the same 1,200 calories? A 150-pound person would need to do 3 hours of aerobics, treadmill or cycling at moderate pace to burn the same amount of calories, or 4 hours of weight training, since weight training burns up to 300 calories per hour or more based upon intensity. So, simple activities around the house can improve your activity level, increase the amount of calories you are expending, and can keep you from being sequestered in a gym for hours at a time.

Another key to becoming less sedentary is to find activities that you will actually do more than once. If you hate running, it would make no sense to prepare for a marathon. One lap around the local track and you'll find yourself at Dairy Queen ordering a Blizzard not knowing how you even got there - or maybe that's just me.

Start with what you like to do and then set goals you can stick with. Not the unachievable and intimidating but rather the simple and the do-able. If you enjoy yard work, then plant a garden or flowers around your yard. Take classes through continuing education programs in your area. They offer activities such as dancing, yoga or other fun stuff that you may feel more comfortable taking than in a regular gym.

Society assumes that overweight people are lazy because we don't see them doing outdoor activities. They don't realize that even if an overweight person is out exercising, they will be made fun, mocked and made embarrassed for exercising in public. A lot of overweight people don't attend gyms or other types of activities because they are either ashamed or they fear being shamed. Richard Simmons has often shared that he began exercising by dancing to music in his room as a teenager, because he didn't want to be made fun of for trying to exercise. Increasing activities around the home will be a great start to becoming more active. As you build confidence, you can expand to more public activities such as going to the park or gym to become even more fit. Here are a few tips to help you burn more calories in your daily life:

10 Tips To Becoming More Active

- Park a little further away from the store or workplace and walk the rest
- Get on or off the bus a block or two from your destination and walk
- Take stairs instead of elevators when you have the option
- Turn off the television and take a walk with your spouse, kids, friend or pet
- Turn on music and dance like no one is watching
- Make time for picnics on weekends and play Frisbee in the park
- Exercise while watching TV (i.e. walk in place, do sit ups, push ups)
- Play outside with your children
- Start a garden; grow healthy vegetables or beautiful flowers, or both!
- Increase physical activity around the house (rake leaves, mow lawn, wash car and hey, maybe even do windows). You'll be fit and have an immaculate home. What a bonus.

Being Fit is a Lifestyle Change

Increasing activity around the house will help you burn more calories and get you started on the right course to fitness. But at some point, a routine is needed to help you achieve your fitness goals. This doesn't mean you need to join a gym, although you may want to, but it does mean that you have to make fitness part of your daily routine. It is all about making it a habit, a part of your lifestyle. I know it may sound overwhelming at first, but you absolutely can do it. And once you start, you won't want to stop. You will love how you feel.

When beginning, you have to put thought into the process of changing your current habits. This is where goal setting comes into play. You don't need to set goals to sleep, shower, or brush your teeth every day. Imagine that, today I'm going to wake up and brush only my bicuspids; tomorrow I will brush my bicuspids and one molar. No, once something is a habit, you just do it. But in order to change your lifestyle into a more active one, you're going to need to set goals and develop a routine. The goals you set need to be challenging yet also obtainable. These goals are for you and only you. They are not goals you can share with a friend or husband or wife. They are unique to your body, your circumstances and your level of physical fitness. You have to really dig deep and evaluate yourself. What are you really willing to do every day? Don't answer with what you would want to do or wish you could do someday.

I knew someone who was very overweight and had an extremely inactive lifestyle. She made a decision to get healthy. The first thing she did was set a goal. She decided walking would be the safest and best exercise for her. She put on her workout clothes, drove to the gym, and walked on the treadmill for a total of one minute. No, she didn't faint or drop dead. She didn't stop to go get a cheeseburger, either. (There's our weight bias kicking in.) She stopped at one minute because that was her goal; to get dressed, go to a gym and walk on the treadmill for exactly one minute. She was proud of herself, as she should have been. She then set a goal to walk two minutes on the treadmill the next day.

To you or me this may seem futile, but to her it was life altering. After only three weeks, she was walking on the treadmill 20 minutes a day. Now she is setting goals for weight lifting and group classes. By setting goals she could obtain, she gained confidence and stamina and is now reaping the benefits of better health. If she initially set a goal to go to the gym to walk for 20 minutes and lift some weights, she could have injured herself or felt overwhelmed and quit the entire idea of exercising. The tortoise is usually the winner of the race.

I did the same thing with vegetables. For the longest time, I would not eat vegetables. In fact, I remember when I was younger George Bush Sr. banned broccoli from the White House. I thought, hey what's good for the White House in Washington is good enough for me here in Queens. So I too decided to ban all the vegetables I hated. However, when I decided to make fitness a part of my lifestyle, I decided this had to change. So I added one vegetable a week to my diet. Instead of filling a grocery cart of every vegetable that existed, I chose to try one new veggie per week. Now I still don't like brussels sprouts very much, but some veggies such as snow peas, carrots, cauliflower, asparagus and leafy spinach have become staples in my diet.

Your next step is to get yourself into a routine. If you have difficulty doing this, then find a workout partner. I am well aware that getting yourself to stick to an activity everyday can be tedious and even boring. This is where a fitness buddy comes in handy. While you both don't have to be at the same fitness level, it is beneficial to find someone that is close to your level so you can both be successful and help each other improve. Find a friend, neighbor, co-worker or someone in your community that you can count on to be consistent with the activity. Your spouse is your spouse - as romantic as it may seem, don't expect him or her to be your fitness buddy too. It is way too easy for excuses to be made; the kids need help with their homework, the boss set deadlines, the dog pooped on the rug, blah, blah, blah. Find someone outside of the home that shares your newfound zeal for fitness. If you know someone is depending on you, then you're much more likely to put on your sneakers and get out of the house.

Below is a chart of activities, which may interest you. Remember finding activities you actually enjoy will make a lifestyle change likely to be permanent. The chart also includes the amount of calories burned for each activity. (All estimates are based on a one-hour session.)

Activity	Weight	Total Approximate Calories Used	Weight	Total Approximate Calories Used
Bicycling	150	450	200	580
Gardening	150	340	200	430
Hiking	150	415	200	550
Mowing lawn/ Push mower	150	325	200	430
Spinning class	150	475	200	635
Stair Climbing	150	610	200	820
Swimming	150	605	200	800
Tennis	150	550	200	730
Walking /Pushing a stroller	150	300	200	395
Walking/ Brisk pace	150	395	200	530
Weight Lifting	150	465	200	625
Yoga	150	360	200	480

I stress start at your own level and listen to your body. You didn't get out of shape in a week and you won't reverse that trend in a week, either. Make changes that will last for a lifetime. This isn't some Get-Fit-Quick scheme. When fitness becomes part of your lifestyle, then it is easier to maintain. For example, instead of watching television in the evening, I started taking my dog for a walk. Now I'm a part of a dog-walking group in my neighborhood.

I have a neighbor who actually does a Boot Camp class at her home three mornings a week. She rustles up a group, they pay a professional trainer to come over to the house and they work out together. It's very cost effective;

they don't have to pay gym membership fees, save money on gas, plus they get the added benefit of group support. The most important part of fitness is finding activities that you enjoy doing. It may take some time to find those activities and it may take you some time to build up a higher level of fitness. But, what else are you going to do? In 5 years you are going to be 5 years older, so why not be 5 years older and fit? Think about the brave lady who started one minute at a time. Put your fears behind you and take the first step of your new journey.

The Incredible Bulk

If you're a woman you may be thinking, "But I don't want to look bulky." If you are overweight, then yes I understand you don't want to appear any larger than you already are. However, there is a difference between body fat and muscle. Building bulk is something that usually worries women - at least I don't know many men who fear putting on too much muscle. In fact, men spend a lot of money, time, and energy trying to build muscle bulk. I find it ironic that women are trying to be stick thin while men are always trying to be the incredible hulk.

Muscle hypertrophy (getting bigger muscles) is very difficult for women since they only produce a small amount of testosterone, which is responsible for muscle growth. Men produce forty to sixty times more testosterone than women. So a woman's chance of getting bulky from working out is about the same as running into Brad Pitt working as the McDonald's drive-thru cashier.

As we all try to become fit, we are looking for that "toned" look that comes from having built some muscle on your frame. This gives us a fit appearance, not an emaciated death look. The more lean body mass you have, the higher your metabolism (burning more fat while at rest). So by missing out on the benefits of weight training, you'll most likely become even fatter, skinny-fat or prone to osteoporosis. If you still want to continue exercising without weight training, and continue your impossible mission for a toned body, good luck to you. But if you are ready to make the leap, here are a few tips to remember:

- Consult with your physician before beginning any training program especially if you have a medical condition such as diabetes or high blood pressure, are overweight, sedentary, over 35 years old or have any heart problems.
- In the beginning, exercise should be limited to an easy pace and exertion. Perhaps some gentle stretching is all you will be able to do initially. No Pain No Gain was invented by some workout nut in the 60's. Stay away from pain!
- Be sure to warm up properly before exercising, such as walking in place for 3 to 5 minutes.
- For cardio, do short workouts, like 2-10 minute sessions rather than longer sessions if you find them too difficult initially.
- Consistency is the key to any fitness program. Do not skip your workouts.
- Cut back if you feel pain. You might feel some soreness at first, but it shouldn't be painful.
- Find a workout partner; this will keep you motivated and accountable.

If you are still hesitant about weight training, then do some research and find a trainer or studio that specializes in working with an overweight population. You don't need the trainer at the gym who feels the need to yell, scream or embarrass people because he is "motivating" them. Make sure they have earned degrees and they aren't untrained individuals who've purchased an online certification from the *Be Healthy by Bert* training program. I enjoy driving a car but considering I know nothing about them, you would never want me to work on your transmission or give you lessons on changing your oil—unless, of course, you like the increased calorie expenditure that comes with tapping your feet to the rhythm of knocking under the hood.

Work Out According To Your Shape

By now you should be on fire to start your new lifestyle. You have a handle on how to be more active and how to eat better. You may be feeling so good you might want to step it up a notch. Let's start by learning training tips based on your body shape so that you can customize your workouts. As you know, you can't change your body type or body shape. However, any body shape can be both unfit and fat or can be fit and healthy. Here are a few strategies to help you based upon your body shape:

Banana Shape Training Tips:

- Build muscle mass through resistance exercise.
- To ensure that you build a symmetrical body shape, all of the muscle groups should be emphasized in both the lower and upper body.
- 2-3 days per week of lifting weights, moderate to heavy with lower reps
- Perform cardio activities to help maintain shape.
- Do at least 3 days of cardio training at moderate intensity for 30 minutes.

Pear Shape Training Tips:

- Focus on exercises that will balance out the top half of your body with the bottom half of your body.
- Do aerobic activities that target the lower body, and resistance exercises for the upper body. This will tone upper body and slim lower body for better symmetry.
- Don't focus too much weight training on lower body. This is often a tendency because the pear shape is strong in lower body. Remember you want balance.
- Do at least three 30-minute cardio sessions per week.
- Do at least two weight-training sessions per week for the upper body.

Apple Shape Training Tips:

- Focus on aerobic training in order to slim down and lose body fat.
- By working on the lower half of your body, you can help balance out your chest and shoulders (but do train upper body as well).
- Do low resistance exercises with lots of repetitions, such as stair climbing, running and incline walking to help balance out the lower body while slimming down the midsection.

- Do at least three 30-40 minute cardio sessions per week.
- Do at least 2-3 workouts per week, total body.
- Focus on the lower body to achieve balance.

Hour Glass Shape Training Tips:

- Focus on both cardio and resistance exercises.
- Cardio will assist in keeping your weight in check, while resistance exercises will help to maintain balance between your upper and lower body.
- Vary your repetitions and keep your resistance weights light so as not to build too much muscle mass.
- Do at least two days of weight training focusing on the lower and upper body.
- Do at least 3 days of cardio at 30 minutes per session.

Just as bodies come in all shapes and sizes, workouts can also be adapted to help each body shape reach its fitness potential. One of the greatest benefits of weight training for all women is that it helps in the prevention of osteoporosis. Studies show that strength training over a period of time can help prevent bone loss and may even help build new bone. If you don't want to be Ms. Hunchback of Notre Dame at 65 years old, start weight training while you're young. Look at it this way - we've all had our share of dating dumbbells, now it's time to lift them.

Blame It On The Bad Diet

It may be possible to look bulky if you eat excessive amounts of food but weight training and muscle mass is not to be blamed. It's a bad diet that is to blame for that "bulky" look. Even when on a regular workout routine, you still need to eat healthy in order to reach your fitness goals. You can't out train a bad diet. Women who choose to lift weights while following a good diet and committed cardio program end up achieving firm looking bodies. The truth is that regardless of your body shape you can sculpt a tone body. Eat for fitness, not thinness. Train, get toned and make skinny scared of you.

Some of you may have children or jobs that limit the amount of time you have to work out. Good news; did you know that mini-workouts – 10 minutes three times a day – are just as effective as a continuous 30-minute workout, according to the American College of Sports Medicine. So, this may mean there are times when you only get 10 to 20 minutes of exercise in per day, but if consistent over the course of the week it will still give you benefits. Shorter workouts, along with a good eating program, can get you in the best shape ever and still allow time for that crazy little thing called life.

To Kill a Scale

Dieting has always been about the daily showdown with the bathroom scale. And usually it is a losing battle in the end. There is an inherent problem with the scale. It doesn't know what it is weighing. When you get on a scale, it measures your body; both fat and lean mass. The scale has no way of differentiating between your liver, lungs, brain, spleen and the fat in your thighs. The scale doesn't know if you have added 5 pounds of muscle or added hair extensions. It can't distinguish between the 3 pounds of body fat you have lost and the 5 pounds of muscle you have gained. So, it simply tells you that you have gained 2 pounds. You get depressed about the 2 pounds you think have gained, rather than rejoicing because you have improved your body composition by 8 pounds.

What is body composition? It is the percentage of body fat and lean body mass (being muscle, bone and organs). This method of measurement is much different than the scales, height-weight charts, or body mass index (BMI) measurements. Body composition measures the difference between body fat and lean body mass, so it gives you a more accurate reflection of your health than the scale. As we have seen with the height weight chart, Arnold Schwarzenegger is considered obese even though he has a very low body fat percentage. Schwarzenegger obese? Please - his abs have abs, and those abs have biceps.

What does this mean to us? Throw your scale out the window, that's what it means. (Oh, how I always wanted someone to say that to me.) Toss it - bang it over and over again with a hammer. Why? Once you start training you're going to see the scale move up, not down. And who needs that right now? You see, you are gaining muscle mass (which will just show up as weight on that dumb old scale). And I don't want this to discourage you or hinder your motivation to move forward. It is actually a fabulous thing that's happening. You want to gain muscle mass because muscle helps burn fat; it helps with posture, gives you increased energy and improves overall health.

Did you get rid of your scale yet? Can't bring yourself to put it in the garbage? Then smother it in a blanket and hide it in the trunk of your car. Call it a few choice bad words while you're at it. Maybe I've been watching too many mobster movies, but go ahead. Do it. Come back when you're done. I'll wait...

Wasn't that fun? Are you smiling yet? Are you feeling like Tony Soprano?

That scale was never a valid means of measurement, so good riddance! When you relied only on that scale, you may not have noticed that your clothes fit looser in your waist, or that you have more energy. You might not have recognized that your back or knees felt better, or that you have a better outlook on life. You might not have recognized the improvements you are making, simply because you have been giving it so much of your power.

Now that the scale is out of your life, let's gain weight - lean body weight, that is. Most likely it was one of the reasons why your diets never worked. You were losing muscle mass and the scale was giving you positive reinforcement for a very bad situation. You were probably not losing any fat at all. Ultimately, the scale made you worse off than if you have never dieted in the first place. Now it's time for your scale to die-t. And time for you to gain—confidence and lean weight.

Get Measured

If you really want to know how fit you are, get your body composition checked. Go to an individual who knows how to take the measurement accurately. Most fitness centers have someone on staff that can perform the measurement or you can contact a local college or hospital.

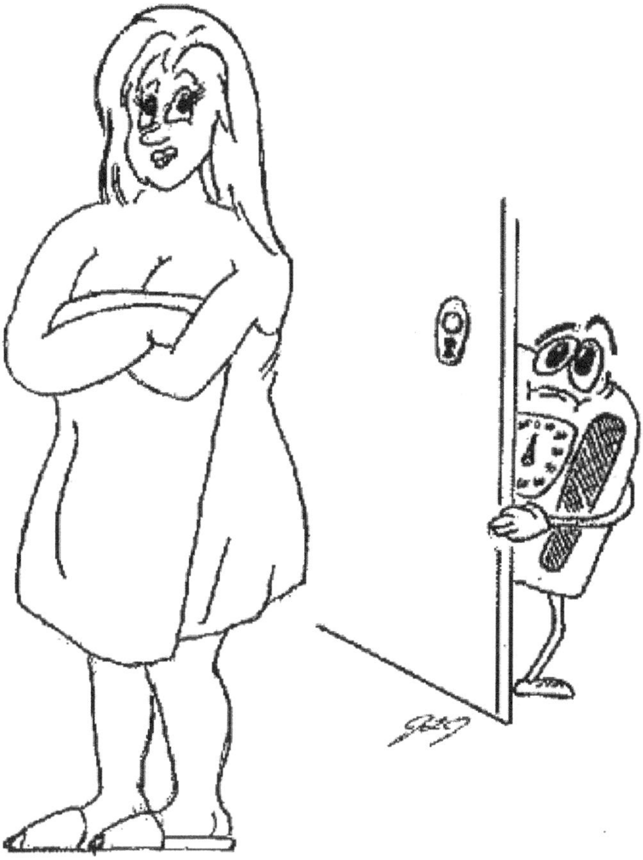

"Hmm, I'm gonna have to change those locks."

They can also help you in setting a realistic goal based upon your current body composition. Calipers are one of the best methods due to both accessibility and cost. I would be cautious about the computers that are used to measure body composition (like Bio Impedance) because they tend to be less accurate if certain rules about water and carbohydrate intake aren't followed beforehand. In case you were wondering, the average adult body fat is approximately 18-24 percent for men and 25-32 percent for women.

Body fat percentage is a much more accurate reflection of overall health, but even it has its limitations. It can't tell you where the fat is stored exactly. And, as we learned earlier, where body fat is stored is just as important as your amount of body fat. If it is stored in the vital organs, it is more harmful than if it is stored under the skin. Even though body fat percentage has its limitations, getting measured is the best way to go in order to get an accurate read of your body and health.

No Such Thing as Spot Reduction

Have you seen the advertisements for the ab blaster? It guarantees that you will have rock hard abs in just minutes a day. There is also the ab roller, ab glider, ab circle and even the ab rocket. (No, the later doesn't shoot you into outer space.) But what is does do, what they all do, is promise you the washboard abs you've only had in your wildest midnight fantasies.

How many millions of these machines do you think have been sold? How many of them do you think have become a clothing rack or part of a garage sale? I must admit that I too have been suckered, I mean compelled into buying one of these contraptions. These types of machines are really no different than fad diets. Every few months a company will offer up the latest and greatest ab machine, which offer you rock hard abs in minutes a day. When it doesn't work there will be another along in a few more months, sometimes by the same company, only this time their product is *new and improved.* Why couldn't they get it right the first time? In reality, the only weight lost is from your wallet, when you give them the fifty bucks to order the damn thing.

Here is the flaw with these machines. You can't focus on one body part for fat loss, which is called spot reduction. That is simply the idea that if you work a specific muscle group you will decrease the amount of fat in that area. The most common example of this is people who focus on abdominal exercises in an effort to lose weight in their stomach. "Spot reduction is a mythical concept that encourages fat loss in a specific area or muscle group on the body," fitness expert Lewis-McCormick explains. "Fat is lost throughout the body in a pattern dependent on genetics, sex, hormones and age."

Overall body fat must be reduced in order for you to lose fat in any particular area.

Basically this means you can do a hundred sit ups every night and it isn't going to make you lose body fat from your stomach. Body fat is stored throughout the body, and stored body fat is used for energy. The body can't isolate the cells from which to take the energy. For example, if you are working abdominals, the body won't use energy just from stored fat in the abdominals. In fact, when you begin to lose body fat you will see it all over your body. It may look like one area is losing fat quicker, but that is only because it had less stored fat. For instance, if you are pear shaped and you store fat in your hips and thighs, then your hips and thighs will seem like the last place you lose fat simply because more is stored there. However, fat is pulled from every fat cell when it is used for energy.

This doesn't mean you shouldn't train your abdominals. You should because they are a muscle group and the more toned they become, the better they look when body fat is decreased. But spending hours trying to burn fat specifically from the abdominals is not going to work. There are other trouble spots such as the back of the arms, which are also targeted by the fitness industry as well. Unfortunately, any promise to spot reduce any area is not just dishonest - it is playing on the insecurities of women everywhere, which is downright shameful.

So please don't fall for fad spot reduction gimmicks. Most of the weight loss industry is nothing but gimmicks. Do you really want your health to be based upon schemes and deceptions? Focus on what really works. Getting a fitness plan together and sticking with it will eventually shape the body you have into a work of beauty. In the end (no pun intended), you have to be the one that is happy with yourself.

The Final Rep, We're Taking It Home

So now that you're doing what you need to do to make yourself healthy and happy, you just may realize that by achieving optimal health, you are also benefiting your family, loved ones and friends. But even beyond your personal relationships, we can look towards an even greater good. What motivates me to continue improving my fitness, besides my own health, is to train for charitable causes. Many schools have Relays for Life that help cancer patients, there are also events for specific causes like during Breast Cancer Awareness Month. Do this with a group of friends and motivate each other to train for one of these beneficent events. What a perfect way to give back to your community and get yourself healthy at the same time. Home is where charity begins, in more ways than one.

Weighing In

Women, for the most part, are communicative creatures. We do things together - we shop together, we do Cosmo quizzes together, we even go to the bathroom together. So, if training is not something you can motivate yourself to do, then why not exercise together. Use a local pool for water aerobics; find a walking trail or even a field where you can gather. I know a 67 year old lady who gets up every morning and walks in a park near her house with her cousin who is 65 years old. They have lost a total of 20 lbs in less than 2 months by simply being consistent with their walking. Their goal is to be healthy, not skinny. But as you get fit, excess weight doesn't hang around. No gyms, weight rooms, or spot reduction gadgets - just two mothers enjoying a walk together every morning, along with their friendship and their fitness.

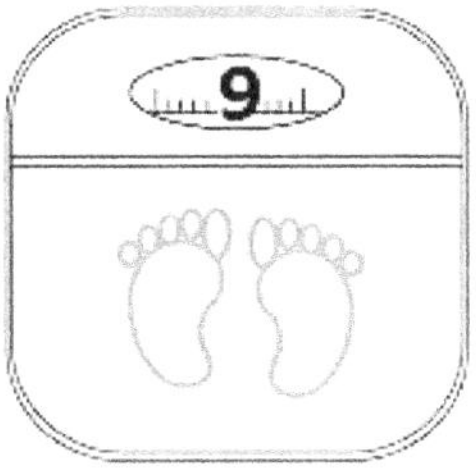

Think Like a Man

I know what you're probably saying to yourself, "Think like a man? But men rarely do think." Ha ha, now that we've had our moment of juvenile joviality, let's put this in perspective. When it comes to weight and dieting, men actually have a healthier view of themselves. They look at their bodies as tools, rather than tying self-worth to their weight. Studies show males are more inclined to action than thinking. And it is in this very difference that we can learn from our male counterparts' behavior. While women are more likely to plan out and think things through, forecasting nearly every possible scenario, men just get started. They "Git R Done" as Larry the Cable Guy ever so ineloquently says in his signature catchphrase.

You know what I like about the way men think? Men don't like to be thought of as skinny. They like to be thought of as lean or muscular. And you know what else I like about the way they think? Most men don't like skinny women either. Isn't that grand? Well-rounded women everywhere should adopt men's well-rounded way of thinking about their well roundedness!

Men Are Not Defined By Their Weight

Men are from Mars, women are from Venus - catchy little phrase, huh? Not only are we worlds apart in the way we express ourselves in relationships, we are worlds apart when it comes to weight. You won't hear a guy say, "Do these jeans make my ass look fat?" Guys don't wake up every morning, step on the scale and cry. The scale doesn't have as much power over them. Usually the only thing a man does with the scale is trip over it, or he may weigh his 25-pound dumbbells to see if they really weigh 25 pounds.

The fact is men and women view their bodies very differently. Women place high value and much of their self worth on how they look and how much they weigh. Men, on the other hand, don't see weight as much more than a number. Studies show that men base their self-worth largely on their productivity, income and stature in the community. Women base their self worth mainly on their body, their sex appeal, and whether or not a man loves them.

One interviewee echoed this sentiment as she explained, "I think men have a different attitude about their bodies than women do. When a woman feels unhappy with her body, she takes it so personally, and she loses so much self-confidence. She relates her worth to how she feels about her body. Even now, I still struggle with it myself...Men see it as a tool, so they eat and workout and don't worry about it so much. Men separate their self worth from their body, but women seem to associate their self worth with their body. Men generally have a wider window of weight that is permissible because of their taller and larger frames. Women are generally smaller and have less weight that they can gain to look overweight."

Often, women are harder critics on themselves and even on other women because we have been conditioned to think we must be thin. Yet the average guy who is overweight may still be seen as strong or manly. Football players or power lifters may be overweight or even obese, but they are seen as real men. They can also be perceived as hardworking, funny, sexy, charming, intelligent and carefree if they are overweight.

Women are defined by their weight because society demands they adhere to a certain beauty standard. When women do not naturally fit the standard or do not constantly strive to fit the standard, they are considered to have failed themselves, and most often are told that they should be ashamed. What is the standard defined by our culture today? Half of women wear a size 14 or larger, but most standard clothing outlets cater to sizes 14 or smaller. Basically the fashion industry is telling most women they are not beautiful. And this simply is not true.

Did you know the average woman weighs 169 pounds? But we don't see this as average because it is portrayed in the media as large and excessive. Women in our culture are expected to be small and dainty, not to take up personal space. Larger women are not seen as objects of sexual desire. For the most part, they are not even taken seriously. Studies show they make less money, are less likely to date and are seen as having no control or discipline. A large size is reflective of power, so women are expected to remain small and fragile so as to be less powerful than their male counterparts. The irony is that large women aren't necessarily seen as powerful, but are invisible to others and usually go unnoticed in society. For the most part, the only time they are acknowledged is in a negative manner, whether they endure discrimination of some type or are made fun of because of their size.

While women of all ethnicities feel a connection between their weight and self-worth, studies suggest that this connection is greatest among white females. A university study, led by Natalie Cole, suggests that white women who base their self-worth on body weight, experience a significant drive toward thinness, despite having healthy body mass indices. Women of other races share a similar, though less significant connection between self-worth and body weight.

This is likely due to the fact that many of the images in advertisements, magazines and the media are of white women, so they experience more pressure to be thin. Women see those objectified images and really identify with that and think, in order to be seen as sexy, they need to look a certain way. While African American, Asian Americans and Hispanic American women may also base their self-worth on weight and are susceptible to dieting behaviors, research shows they don't typically face the same pressure. The exception here is when they are placed in the spot light due to certain levels of success. For example, women like Oprah Winfrey, Jennifer Lopez and Tyra Banks face tremendous pressures to be thin.

Women experience a much greater bias than do men. We need to start changing that way of thinking. It has always been acceptable for a man to have a beer gut or be a "bear." We find that cozy, cute and endearing. But if we are overweight we consider ourselves disgusting, gross and worthless. This is because the media and fashion industry has conditioned women, especially Caucasian women, to link their self-worth to their weight - or rather their lack of weight. It's not that men aren't held up to certain beauty standards (or handsome standards, you could call them), it's just that a woman's value is based so much more on how she looks than what she does. Do you really think most men care what anyone, including society thinks about their physique? Not really, so why do you place so much pressure on yourself? The irony is that men care less about how we look than other women.

Men see their bodies as an instrument they work with in order to get things done in life. So you need to think of the awesome things your body can do. Only a woman can carry life for nine months and give birth to a newly created human being. Only a woman can breastfeed. Only a woman can be a grandmother, a sister, an aunt, a wife. Only a woman can be, well...a woman. And all the amazing things that come with womanhood. Your body is a wonderful and impressive tool. Appreciating your body as such may not stop you from having a few "I feel fat" days, but it will help you put them into a more healthy perspective.

Feed Your Ego

Women are just as competitive as guys, but our ego isn't as tied to how fast we run or what we bench-press. Maybe it should be! Ego is a powerful motivator. The next time you have an amazing workout, brag—even if to yourself. When you experience success by finally doing things the right way, you will feel a sense of pride and accomplishment. Sometimes a big part of the problem is that you haven't felt successful in a long time. So celebrate your achievements, don't downplay them.

Work ethic, competition and ego are attributes often associated with males, but they can be attributed to women as well. Research shows that female students who participate in sports have higher self-esteem, perform better in school and are more likely to be successful in college. This is because these traits have been instilled in them at a young age. These females focus on goals and accomplishments to feed their self-worth, rather than on their body shape.

Be Realistic

Men are not typically perfectionists. "Most guys avoid anything that even smacks of perfectionism," and that applies to dieting too, says *Prevention* advisor Pamela Peeke, MD, an assistant clinical professor of medicine at the University of Maryland School of Medicine. "When women start a diet, they go from zero to 100, they want to become perfect overnight, which is a hallmark of failure. That's why I developed the 80% rule: Hit your weight loss goals 80% every single day you can. One day, it'll be 100% because it happens to be a great day. Other days, you'll hit 50% because life tosses a curve ball."

A recent Auburn University study found that women feel inadequate at home and at work more often than men because women are more perfectionistic. Men tend to be risk takers, so they accept that they may fall flat sometimes. Women often care more about what others think than if they achieved a goal. Women tend to only feel good about themselves when every aspect of their lives is going well. Why do we put such unrealistic expectations on ourselves? It is time to realize we aren't perfect, no one is or ever was perfect, and that having an expectation of perfection will only lead to continued failure and disappointment in every area of life.

A Donut is Just a Donut

We know that food can be addictive physically and emotionally. When you come home after a hard day, it's easy to reach for the bag of cookies or donuts. However, a donut is just a donut. It isn't going to make your problems go away. Generally, men see food as food. It is fuel to them. While my comfort food is more likely to be salty pretzels or double-chocolate chip ice cream, my husband's comfort food is a thick, juicy steak. A Cornell University study found that women seek out sweets to ward off the blues but men turn to meat when they want to indulge.

Why does this give him a weight loss advantage? He's eating protein, which will help fill him up (and curb overeating later) far better than any coffee crumb cake would.

One study found that women binge eat more than men do. And when emotions (not your stomach or brain) drive choices, it's a diet disaster. Treat food as fuel. Take bites because you're hungry or need energy, not because of stress or boredom. Think about what your choices will do for your health and let yourself indulge occasionally, halting the guilt. When you eat a donut, don't think, "Oh donuts are my weakness," or you will feel guilty. Think of it simply as a tasty treat and then move on!

What's interesting is that men typically don't munch on things like 100-calorie snack packs. In fact, research shows men are less likely to eat goods labeled *diet* or *low-cal.* And that's actually better for them because they get more nutrients and avoid sneaky saturated fat by fueling up on whole foods, which are also more psychologically filling. When you're hungry, reach for foods such as nuts, turkey, cheese sticks, fruit and vegetables rather than those cute, little low-cal snack packs.

Pump Iron

As your fitness level increases, don't be afraid to start lifting weights. Only about 17% of women do strength training, but did you know that it revs up the metabolism, torches calories and sculpts sexy muscles. It's so effective that I recommend you eventually split your exercise time between cardio and strength training 50-50. As your strength training improves, spend less time on machines and embrace free weights, especially barbells, which work more muscles. As we've learned, the muscle that you are gaining weighs more than the fat you are losing - you may not drop pounds, but you'll be firmer and fit. This is important because as women age, they actually lose muscle mass. Without proper strength training, women lose about half a pound of muscle per year beginning in their mid to late 20's. By the time you are in your 40's, you may have lost up to 10 pounds of muscle.

When you increase muscle mass, you also increase your metabolism. In fact, for every pound of muscle you gain, your body will burn 15-25 more calories per day. This means if you gain four pounds of muscle, you will burn an extra 100 calories per day. You can actually increase your caloric intake because you will be burning more calories. Who wouldn't want that? You can actually eat more food because you are gaining more sexy muscles.

As your fitness improves and you develop a regular strength-training program, drop the Barbie weights. If you're doing two sets of 12 or 15 reps, your weights are probably too light. Move toward higher poundage that makes you strain to do 8 to 10 reps. Once your body is used to 10, then increase the weight until you're only able to do 4-6 reps. Interestingly, expert Lou Schuler says, "At sports medicine conferences, I've seen scans of women's upper arms before and after this kind of training program, and the girth of their upper arms hasn't changed, but you can see the fat tissue is reduced and how much more muscle there is." I say we pump up the volume while we pump ourselves some iron.

Set Performance Goals

Men may be genetically geared toward specific goals. In the beginning (not the Book of Genesis, more like the Chronicles of the Caveman) the male species were the hunters, which meant they were very focused on hunting their game. When they went out to hunt T-Rex, nothing else mattered to them. In order to survive, they set their sights on a goal and attacked it, if you will. The female of our species were the gatherers, which meant they were more multi-task oriented. They had to gather food, firewood, take care of the children and then cook the meat that was killed and brought back from the hunt.

Fast-forward to modern day society and some of these traits still exist. Women are prone to multitasking, so they often don't set specific goals. This is especially true when it comes to their health. Women tend to care for others; it is in their nature. I'm asking you to channel your inner caveman - set your sights on a goal and attack it. Hone in on **your** health and make it a priority. You can do this by setting performance goals.

What men tend to do, which many women don't, is supplement their look-better goals with performance-based ones. In other words, although Roger Federer's physique may be a long-term target, a guy will also set out to do 10 more squats than last week. Approaching a workout this way—naming specific performance goals rather than seeing your session only as a means to a tighter rear end—makes you more successful, says Mark Anshel, Ph.D., a professor of health and human performance at Middle Tennessee State University. Why? You are engaged and have something achievable to strive for during each workout. And because goals constantly change, you get to revel in mini-successes over and over, versus waiting and waiting for the scale to budge.

Benchmarks push you to try harder in the moment, which translates to a harder body later. Studies show that when a woman's mind-set is moved away from the scale and she is challenged, for example to add 10 pounds to her squat, she trains more effectively. Knowing this, I will be certain to make performance goals apart of my daily work out routine. Other than his need to be naked all the time, the caveman has nothing on me.

Empowerment Begins Within

As the great American businesswoman Mary Kay Ash once said, "If you think you can, you can. And if you think you can't, you're right." There was a survey taken in California in which one of the questions was: If you felt really secure about your body, would you stay in the job or relationship that you are in now? Many of the women replied no, they would not. This reinforces the notion that a woman's self worth is intricately tied to how she feels about her body. Are you so self-conscious that you refuse to try new things? Do you feel like you deserve the life you have because you've been conditioned to think that way? So many women let others define them and put them in a box from which they can't seem to escape. If you have children, you are a mom. If you are married, you are so and so's wife. If you are beautiful, that becomes a description of who you are. There isn't anything wrong with any of those associations, but there is so much more to you than just any one part of your life.

Empowerment is about realizing your potential and then pursuing it with vigor. Empowerment is an attitude, as well. Think of the male ego. Whether they are driven by ego or healthy self-esteem, lots of the guys I know believe they're doing great and rarely doubt their ability to succeed, even in the face of setbacks. Even female athletes become distraught or beat themselves up if they don't notice results right away. Ban disempowering thinking! Keep telling yourself that not every day will be a winner but that you *will* win at healthy weight loss. A donut overdose or skipped workout doesn't mean failure. Understand that your next meal will be back on track or your workout tomorrow will be a good one. I promise you'll love your results at the finish line.

I have a fond memory of taking a group of middle school students to Disney World. I was in charge of the seventh grade girls. (After my previous day with the teenage boys, I was looking forward to a much quieter day with the girls.) How wrong I was! They raced around the park with what seemed to be boundless energy, riding the attractions multiple times. It was when we arrived at MGM Studio's Rock 'n' Roller Coaster that a fond memory was born. As the Aero Smith song Dude Looks Like a Lady played, the girls were enthusiastically singing along, their words being most indisputably Do it Like a Lady. When I asked them what they were saying, they all insisted the words were do it like a lady. Their argument was, and I quote, "It's a song about girls doing things better than boys because we usually do." I thought to myself, what a wonderful display of self–esteem. They understand that they are in control of their lives and no one else.

They understand that women can do whatever they set their sights on and yes, they can even do things better than the guys, if they so choose. It was one of those teachable moments except I was the one being taught. They continued to sing their version of the song the rest of the day. It's been 10 years and when I hear that song, it always brings a smile to my face. I think of the mindset of that group of teenage girls. How blessed they were to be in an environment with parents that didn't set limits for them and teachers that empowered them to believe they could do anything and become anything they desired. They came in all shapes and sizes. Some would be considered overweight, but they didn't feel different because they weren't treated differently. That is my vision for all of you reading this now. Whether you are doing it like a lady or thinking like a man, you can become anything you dream and desire to be with planning and hope. Whether it is losing weight, changing careers, improving relationships, starting a family, moving to a new city, we all need our own version of the Do It Like a Lady song so we, too can enthusiastically sing on life's Rock 'n' Roller Coaster.

Permit yourself to realize your abilities. Think and step outside of the box that people have put you. You have many more goals to achieve than you think you have right now. Here are a few practical thoughts in helping you get to where you want to go:

Tips for Empowerment:

- **Believe in Yourself**: Don't be critical of your body or your failures. Thinking negatively about yourself is one of the greatest causes of limitation in life.
- **Love Yourself**: If you don't love yourself, you can't fully love others.
- **Take Control of Your Health**: It's hard to feel empowered when you are unhealthy.
- **Discover and Use Your Talents**: Your passions are often your talents. Cultivate them to their fullest potential.
- **Remember, a Higher Power Helped Make You Who You Are**: In this realm of thought, nothing is impossible, so never settle for less than your best effort, knowing that divine blessings abound.
- **Think, Plan, and Prepare. Be proactive, not reactive:** This will position you to be in more control in any situation you may find yourself.
- **Balance Your Relationships**: Whether married or dating, make sure you are in relationships that are balanced and relationships where you feel equal.

- **Don't Take Life Too Seriously**: After all the planning and hard work, don't forget to relax, laugh hard at yourself. Remember, laughter is cheaper than a hospital visit.

Empowerment doesn't mean you will rule the world. You can have control over your life without controlling the world, you know. Your life is a microcosm. So to all the control freaks out there I must say; control your world and maybe, just maybe you will find that you had control over something much bigger in the end. But always remember that control can only start with the person in the mirror. Empowerment begins from within. It means taking time to care for you. Keep in mind, men often do things for themselves. Sometimes a self-sequestering in the "man cave" is probably their secret to keeping relatively sane.

You may always be the one to ensure that everyone else's needs are met (which can leave you feeling exhausted and far from empowered); but with a strong plan, support of good friends and family, you can share your much-endured burdens and still remain confident in your abilities. True empowerment always comes full circle. All roads lead back to you, your health and your wellness. Eat properly, become more active, balance every aspect of yourself, and you will gain the strength and confidence to master your health and your life.

Give yourself authority to take control over your health. Have new eyes and gain new perspective. You control circumstances; there is no victim of circumstance. What we eat and what we choose to do with our time is totally our decision. Commission yourself to be your own advocate. You have all that you need. Now act on it by making choices that will make you stronger and more confident.

Reflections on Blessings

"Reflect upon your present blessings - of which every man has many - not on your past misfortunes, of which all men have some." ~ *Charles Dickens*

A life not examined is not worth living. It is important to take time to reflect on where you are, where you have been and how you can use that knowledge to get where you want to be. If you don't take that time, surely will you continue to do the same things in the hope that life will turn out different. One of the best ways to reflect on blessings is to keep a daily journal. Sure, you can also use it to vent on issues that are bothersome, but ideally I'd prefer you to write a list of the things for which you are grateful. Write down the positive aspects of your life so as to encourage yourself in the pursuit of better health and wellness. We too often focus on our reactionary side and on the undesirable events that have transpired. Life is too short for that, my friend. Write goals for the day, the decade, or even the mission statement for your life. Dream big, but plan in small increments. Buy a beautiful notebook and write in it every morning for ten minutes. Write about the little things we seem to forget or are hesitant to celebrate. See your future by creating it with words and thoughts. Write with vigor, until and you can't write anymore. Here's your chance to welcome joy back into your life.

The Final Weigh In

"When I stand before God at the end of my life, I would hope that I would not have a single bit of talent left and could say, I used everything you gave me." ~ *Erma Bombeck*

Remember that life is, well...life. That means there are no simple answers to problems, there is no perfect body, and there is no getting out if it alive. As you get older, you realize how swiftly life passes by. Do you really want to spend the short time you have here worrying about weighing a certain number on a scale or looking like an actress in a magazine? Do you want life to be filled with disappointment and regret? Do you want media bias to scare you into causing harm to your body? A resounding NO MORE. By allowing the messages in this book to be absorbed into your thoughts and daily actions, you will stop focusing on being thin but rather on becoming healthy and well. Optimal health is not achieving a specific weight, it is about making proactive decisions to improve your eating habits and activity level; it is about improving your emotional, social and spiritual well being.

Take the hand you are dealt and get in the game; maximize your talents and your strengths. Abraham Lincoln once said, “Whatever you are, be a good one.” Don’t look bitterly towards what others have that you may not. You don’t know the struggles they have had to endure to get there. At the stranger’s first glance, my life may seem fun or glamorous, but the one assuming that hasn’t been around throughout the years to know the valleys and mountains that were descended and climbed, usually alone, to get to whom I am today. I am grateful for each and every struggle because through each, I was able to find out a bit more about myself; who I am and what bears meaning in my life.

Embrace your unique differences because what we may perceive as a frailty is often strength in disguise. Step out on faith and see what the world has to offer and what you have to offer the world. It is all so very beautiful.

And in the end, my wish for you dear friend is to find your new beginning.

It is already there within you.

Bibliography

Allon, N. (1982). The stigma of overweight in everyday life In Wolman, B. *Psychological aspects of obesity*. New York: Van Nostrand Reinhold Company.

American Academy of Pedriatrics (2006). Committee on communications. children, adolescents, and advertising, in *Pediatrics* Vol. 118 No. 6 December, p. 2563-2569.

Andersen, A & DiDomenico, L (1992). Diet vs. shape content of popular male and female magazines: A dose-response relationship to the incidence of eating disorders? *International Journal of Eating Disorders* Vol. 11, no. 3,pp. 283-287.

Baillie-Hamilton PF. Chemical toxins: a hypothesis to explain the global obesity epidemic. J Altern Complement Med 8(2):185–192 (2002

Begley, Sharon. Why Chemicals Called Obesogens May Make You Fat.. *Newsweek*. - 11/09/2009.

Berg, F. M. (2004) Underage and overweight: America's childhood obesity crisis-what every family needs to know. New York: Hatherleigh Press.

Botta, R. (1999). Television images and adolescent girls' body image disturbance. *Journal of Communication* V 49 (2) p. 22-41.

Botta, R. (2003). For your health? The relationship between magazine reading and adolescents' body image and eating disturbances. *Sex Roles,* 48 (9-10) p. 389-399.

Bray, G., Nielsen, S., & Popkin, B. (2004*)*. Consumption of high-fructose corn syrup in beverages may play a role in the epidemic of obesity. *American Journal of Clinical Nutrition* 79 p.537-43.

Brownell, K., Puhl, R., Scwartz, M. & Rudd, L. (Eds.). (2005). *Weight bias.* New York: Guilford Press.

Brownell, K. & Horgen, K. (2004) *Food fight: The inside story of the food industry, America's obesity crisis, and what we can do about it.* New York: McGraw-Hill

Campbell, W., Crim, M., Young, V. and Evans, W. 1994. Increased energy requirements and changes in body composition with resistance training in older adults. *American Journal of Clinical Nutrition*, 60: 167-175.

Connolly HM, Crary JL, McGoon MD, et al. *Valvular heart disease associated with fenfluramine-phentermine. N Engl J Med. 1997;337:581–588*

Crawford, D., Jeffery, R., & French, S. (1999). Television viewing, physical inactivity and obesity. *International Journal of Obesity* Volume 23, Number 4, 437-440.

Critser, G. (2003). *Fat land: How Americans became the fattest people in the* world. New York: Houghton Mifflin.

Cutler, D., Glaeser, E., & Shapiro, J. (2003). Why have Americans become more obese? *National Bureau of Economic Research,* Working paper 9446.

Devereux RB. Appetite suppressants and valvular heart disease. N Engl J Med. 1998;339:765–767.

DiMeglio D., Mattes R..(2000). Liquid versus solid Carbohydrate: Effects on food intake and body weight. *Intl J Obes Relat Metab Disord* 2000;24:794–800.

Eisenberg, M., Neumark-Sztainer, D., & Story, M. 2003). Associations of Weight-Based Teasing and Emotional Well-being Among Adolescents. *Archives of Pediatric and Adolescent Medicine.* Vol.157 p.733-738.

Farley, T., & Cohen, D. (2001). Fixing a fat nation: Why diets and gyms won't save the obesity epidemic. *Washington Monthly,* December, 33, 23.

Field, A., Cheung, L., Wolf, A., Herzog, D., Gortmaker, S., Colditz, G. (1999). Exposure to the mass media and weight concerns among girls. *Pediatrics* vol.103 no. 3, p. 36.

Foley, D. Lose Weight Like A Guy. *Prevention Magazine* December 2011.

Friedman, K., Reichmann, S., & Costanzo, P., (2002) Body image partially mediates the relationship between obesity and psychological distress *Obesity Research* 10 p.33-41.

Garine, I. & Pollock, N. (eds.) (1995). *Social aspects of obesity.* New York: Taylor and Francis.

Greenburg, B, Eastin, E., Hofschire, K. et al. (2003). Portrayals of overweight and obese individuals on commercial television *American Journal of Public Health* Aug Vol. 93, No. 8.

Grun and B. Blumberg. "Endocrine Disrupters as Obesogens.." *Mol Cell Endocrinol.* 304 (2009): 19 - 29.

Himes, S. & Thompson, K. (2007). Fat stigmatization in television shows and movies: A content analysis *Obesity Research* 15 p.712-718.

Hurlock, H and Perrine, S. (2010). Fat epidemic linked to chemicals run amok, NBCnews.com

Janelle KC, Barr SI. Nutrient intakes and eating behavior scores of vegetarian and non vegetarian women. *J Am Diet Assoc.* 1995;95:180-189.

Janesick A, Blumberg B. Endocrine disrupting chemicals and the developmental programming of adipogenesis and obesity. Birth Defects Res Part C Embryo Today Rev. 2011;93(1):34–50.

Janesick A, Blumberg B. Minireview: PPARγ as the target of obesogens. J Steroid Biochem Mol Biol 127(1–2):4–8 (2011).

Johnson, Brad. (2008). *Oppression of Obesity.* Retrieved from: *http://eaglescholar.georgiasouthern.edu:8080/jspui/handle/10518/39*

Jollis JG, Landolfo CK, Kisslo J, et al. Fenfluramine and phentermine and cardiovascular findings: effect of treatment duration on prevalence of valve abnormalities. *Circulation. 2000;101:2071–2077.*

Keith, L. (2009) *The Vegetarian Myth: Food, Justice, and Sustainability*. Flash Point Press. Oakland, Ca.

Klaczynski, P. A., Goold, K. W., & Mudry, J. J. (2004). Culture, obesity stereotypes, self-esteem, and the "thin ideal": A social identity perspective. *Journal of Youth and Adolescence, 33*(4), 307.

Klesges, R., Shelton, M., & Klesges, L. (1993). Effects of Television on Metabolic Rate: Potential implications for childhood obesity *Pediatrics* Vol. 91 No. 2 February, pp. 281-286.

Kotz, K., Story, M. (1994). Food advertisements during children's Saturday morning television programming: are they consistent with dietary recommendations? *Journal of the American Dietetic Association.* Nov. (11) p.1296-300.

Latner, J. & Stunkard, A. (2003). Getting worse: the stigmatization of obese children *Obesity Research* 11 p.452-456.

Lea, EJ, Crawford D, Worsley A. Public views of the benefits and barriers to the consumption of a plant-based diet. *EurJ Clin Nutr.* 2006;60:828-37.

Macfarlane BJ, van der Riet WB, Bothwell TH, Baynes RD, Siegenberg D, Schmidt U, Tol A, Taylor JRN, Mayet F. Effect of traditional Oriental soy products on iron absorption. *Am J Clin Nutr.* 1990;51:873-880.

Markowitz, GS, et.al (1998) Acute interstitial nephritis following treatment with anorectic agents phentermine and phendimetrazine. *Clin Nephrol.* Oct;50(4):252-4.

Messina M, Redmond G. Effects of soy protein and soybean isoflavones on thyroid function in healthy adults and hypothyroid patients: a review of the relevant literature. *Thyroid.* 2006;16:249-258.

Nestle, M. (2002*). Food politics.* Los Angeles, Ca.: University of California Press.

O'Brien, R. The Dirty Dozen: 12 Foods Coated in Chemicals *Prevention Magazine June 20, 2012.*

Pierce, J. & Wardle, J. (1997).Cause and effect beliefs and self-esteem of overweight children *Journal of Child Psychology and Psychiatry* 38,p.645-650.

Pikosky, M., Faigenbaum, A., Westcott, W., and Rodriguez, N. 2002. Effects of resistance training on protein utilization in healthy children. *Medicine and Science in Sports and Exercise*, 34 (5): 820-827.

Pratley, R., Nicklas, B., Rubin, M., Miller, J., Smith, A., Smith, M., Hurley, B., and Goldberg, A. 1994. Strength training increases resting metabolic rate and norepinephrine levels in healthy 50 to 65 year-old men. *Journal of Applied Physiology*, 76: 133-137.

Robinson, T., Borzekowski, D., Matheson, D., & Kraemer, H. (2007). Effects of fast food branding on young children's taste preferences. *Archives of Pediatrics & Adolescent Medicine.*161: 792-797.

Schlosser, E. (2001). *Fast food nation.* New York: Houghton Mifflin Co.

Stearns, P. (1997). *Fat History: Bodies and beauty in the modern west.* New York: New York University Press.

Stroebele, N., De Castro, J.(2004). Television viewing is associated with an increase in meal frequency in humans. *Appetite*. Feb.42(1):111-3.

Tang-Péronard JL, et al. Endocrine-disrupting chemicals and obesity development in humans: a review. Obes Rev. 2011;12(8):622–636

Underwood, Ann (December 2011) 7 Foods That Should Never Cross Your Lips Is your food loaded with toxins and chemicals? Here, simple swaps to protect yourself Retrieved from *Prevention Online Magazine*

Villegas R, Gao YT, Yang G, Li HL, Elasy TA, Zheng W, Shu XO. Legume and soy food intake and the incidence of type 2 diabetes in the Shanghai Women's Health Study. *Am J Clin Nutr.* 2008;87:162-167.

Wolfe SM, Sasich LD, Barbenhenn E. Petition to FDA to ban the diet drug sibutramine (Meridia) [HRG publ no 1613]. Washington: US Food and Drug Administration; 2002 Mar 19.

Made in the USA
Monee, IL
04 November 2026

67386408R00085